Latrina Walden™
Exam Solutions



# Psych Medications:

## Common medications

For: NPs, PMHNPs, RNs, LPCs

# Disclaimer



## Legal stuff

Products produced, published or sold by www.latrinawaldenexamsolutions.com including but not limited to blogs, podcasts, courses, digital materials and all other products are for entertainment and informational purposes only and should not be used to make medical diagnosis, give medical advice or prescribe medical treatment.

## More legal stuff

These productions are designed to provide accurate information in regard to the subject matter covered and uses reasonable efforts to ensure that such information is accurate. LWES assumes no responsibility for correctness, accuracy or recommendations in the products or errors omissions or any outcomes related to your use of the products.

## Mandatory legal stuff

LWES products may provide information, guidance and recommendations related to a variety of subject matters, including but not limited to, medical treatment, emergency care, drugs, medical devices and side effects; however research, clinical practice and government regulations often change the accepted standards and is solely your responsibility and not the responsibility of LWES to determine appropriate medical treatment, the use of any drug in the clinical setting, and for determining FDA status of a drug, reading the package insert and reviewing prescribing information for the most up to date recommendations on doe, precautions, and contraindication and determining the appropriate usage for a product.

# Disclaimer



## More legal mandatory stuff

Products are intended solely as a guide and for educational purposes are not intended to be used for actual medical treatment or as a statement of any standard of care. These products are provided as is and is available without warranty whether expressed or implied. You understand that your use of this is at your sole risk.

ISBN 978-1-7369010-4-5

9 781736 901045

# How to Use This Book

## ONLINE COURSE

**There is an accompanying online course to this manual. You do not need it, but it is recommended. This is specifically for those who have visual needs in learning. The online course is separate and can be located at www.latrinawaldenexamsolutions.com**

**If you need help in locating the course contact us and our representative can assist you! Happy studying!**

## WHAT IS THIS COURSE?

**This course is for professionals working in psychiatric nursing or mental health care who require a quick and reliable reference guide to the medications used to treat their patients. Whether you're a Nurse Practitioner, Counselor, RN, LPN, Psychologist, or Psychiatrist, this course will provide essential explanations and insights into the complex and less commonly known medications in the field.**

## WHO IS THIS FOR?

**This book is a psychiatric medication guide designed for those who need a general introduction and quick reference to psychiatric nursing medications. It offers simple, clear explanations of the classification of each medication, their brand names, and key clinical pearls. Additionally, the book provides clinical indications for each medication, giving readers a comprehensive understanding of their use in practice. It's an essential tool for navigating the often complex and lesser-known medications in psychiatric care.**

# Table of Contents

Section 1

# Antidepressants

## Dosage Variations

10 mg, 20 mg, and 40 mg tablets taken once daily, as well as an oral solution with a concentration of 10 mg/5 mL

Antidepressants

# Citalopram (Celexa)

## Mechanism of Action

**Classification: SSRI;** Stimulates Serotonin activity with mild antagonist action on histamine

## Indications

- **MDD (Major Depressive Disorder)**
  - Adults 18+
  -Poorly metabolized in 60+ due to 2C19

  ***Off Label:*** *GAD, SAD, OCD, PD, PTSD, PMDD*

## Pharmacokinetics

- Onset: 1 to 4 weeks
- Half-life elimination: 24 to 48 hours (average, 35 hours)
- Metabolized primarily by CYP450 3A4 and 2C19

## Adverse Effects/Contraindications

1. 40 mg = risk due to QT prolongation
2. Caution pregnancy but Ok for Breastfeeding
3. Hyponatremia from SIADH (rare)
4. May increase risk of bleeding
5. Contraindicated to MAOIs

*Most Common Adverse Effects*

- CNS: Drowsiness, insomnia, dizziness, headache (dose-dependent)
- Dermatologic: Diaphoresis (sweating)
- Gastrointestinal: Nausea, vomiting, xerostomia, constipation, diarrhea, yawning
- Sexual: Ejaculation disorder (impotence) (dose-dependent)

## Pearls

- *Electrolytes, especially potassium and sodium, should be monitored and evaluated*
- *A chance of developing serotonin hyperactivity at therapeutic doses, primarily if using another serotonergic medication concomitantly*
- *Weight and growth should be monitored regularly by a clinician during treatment in children and adolescents (increased risk of suicide in youth so monitor)*

Antidepressants

# Escitalopram (Lexapro)

## Dosage Variations

Orally and is available in 2 forms—an oral solution at a concentration of 1mg/mL and tablets in 5mg, 10mg, or 20mg strengths ( max dose MDD)

## Mechanism of Action

**Classification: SNRI;** Reuptaking serotonin from the synaptic cleft into the presynaptic neuron. Inactivation of SERT by escitalopram leads to an elevation in synaptic serotonin levels i.e. a serotonin reuptake inhibitor

## Indications

- **Generalized Anxiety Disorder (GAD)**

- Beginning at 7+ years old

- **MDD (Major Depressive Disorder) <unipolar>**

- Both acute and maintenance phase
- Adolescents and adults

**Off Label:** SAD, OCD, PD, PTSD, PMDD, vasomotor symptoms of menopause

## Pharmacokinetics

- Food does not affect the absorption of the drug
- Peak plasma time: 5 hours
- Steady-state plasma concentrations within 1 to 2 weeks
- Hepatic metabolism via CYP3A4 and CYP2C19
- Half-life of escitalopram: 27 to 33 hours

## Adverse Effects/Contraindications

- Caution renal and hepatic impairment clients
- Caution pregnancy but Ok for Breastfeeding
- Hyponatremia for 60+ is a risk
- Risk of Serotonin Syndrome
- Risk of QT prolongation
- SSRIs, including escitalopram, inhibit platelet function, thereby elevating the risk of bleeding
- Risk of bleeding also increases when escitalopram is concomitantly administered with NSAIDs
- Undergo regular monitoring for mood or behavioral changes, including signs of suicidality

## Pearls

- *Excreted in your urine*
- *Symptoms of Hyponatremia can vary depending on its severity, ranging from anorexia, nausea, vomiting, fatigue, and headache to more critical conditions such as altered mental status, seizures, and, in extreme cases, coma.*
- *Can potentially exacerbate sinus bradycardia and atrioventricular (AV) block by inhibiting sodium and calcium channels*
- *It is essential to implement measures for maintaining appropriate temperature and blood pressure control*

Antidepressants

# Fluoxetine (Prozac)

## Dosage Variations

Oral solution (20mg/5ml), tablet (10mg, 20mg, 60mg), capsule (10mg, 20mg, 40mg), and delayed release capsule (90mg)

## Mechanism of Action

**Classification (SSRI);** exerts its effects by blocking the reuptake of serotonin into presynaptic serotonin neurons by blocking the reuptake transporter protein located in the presynaptic terminal. Fluoxetine also has mild activity at the 5HT2A and 5HT2C receptors. i.e. serotonin reuptake inhibitor

## Indications

- **Obsessive –Compulsive Disorder (peds)**
- **Panic Disorder**
- **Bulimia**
- **Binge Eating**
- **Premenstrual Dysphoric Disorder**
- **Bipolar Disorder**
- **MDD (Major Depressive Disorder)**
- **- 8 + yrs or older**
- **-Treatment resistant depression with Olanzapine**

## Pharmacokinetics

- Half-life: 2 to 4 days
- Effect emerges within 2 to 4 weeks
- Cytochrome P450 enzyme (CYP2D6)
- Hepatic metabolism via CYP3A4 and CYP2C19
- Half-life of escitalopram varies from 27 to 33 hours

## Adverse Effects/Contraindications

- Breastfeeding is not recommended
- Taper 3rd trimester of pregnancy due to toxic effect to fetus
- Patients may even have a panic attack with the administration of fluoxetine
- Most side effects are immediate and disappear with time. Thus, waiting for the side effects to subside is best before altering treatment.
- When taken in conjunction with alcohol, it may cause ataxia and respiratory depression
- Risk of serotonin syndrome is present
- Should monitor children and adolescent patients for suicidal ideation

## Pearls

- *Longest half-life of SSRI's*
- *decreased weight gain is associated with the administration of fluoxetine in children and adolescent patients*
- *NSAIDs(e.g., ibuprofen) may impair the effectiveness of fluoxetine*
- *fluoxetine should be discontinued five weeks before initiating monoamine oxidase inhibitor therapy to avoid precipitating serotonin syndrome*

Antidepressants

# Paroxetine (Paxil)

## Dosage Variations

Orally administered and can be taken with or without food any time of the day. Given in tablets but also available in controlled-release tablet and liquid form.

## Mechanism of Action

**Classification (SSRI);** Paroxetine's signature mechanism of action is to block the serotonin reuptake transporter (SERT) and thus increase the concentration of synaptic serotonin. Current theory suggests that the diminished serotonin concentration in the depressed brain induces the upregulation of serotonergic receptors.

## Indications

**FDA-approved Indications**

- First-line treatment of major depressive disorder
- Obsessive-compulsive disorder(OCD)
- Panic disorder
- Post-traumatic stress disorder(PTSD)
- Premenstrual dysphoric disorder
- Social Anxiety Disorder (SAD)

**Non-FDA-approved Indications**

- Binge eating disorder
- Body dysmorphic disorder
- Bulimia Nervosa (BN)
- Generalized Anxiety Disorder (GAD)
- Premature ejaculation

## Pharmacokinetics

- Half-life: 2 to 4 days
- Effect emerges within 2 to 4 weeks
- Cytochrome P450 enzyme (CYP2D6)
- Hepatic metabolism via CYP3A4 and CYP2C19
- Half-life of escitalopram varies from 27 to 33 hours

## Adverse Effects/Contraindications

- The primary side effects of sertraline include syncope, lightheadedness, diarrhea, nausea, sweating, dizziness, xerostomia, confusion, hallucinations, tremor, somnolence, impotence, a disorder of ejaculation, fatigue, rhinitis, and female sexual disorder.
- Bleeding may appear as it may inhibit platelet aggregation
- Rarely produce symptoms of serotonin syndrome
- Increase the risk of suicidal ideation and behavior in children, adolescents, and young adults with major depression
- Requires caution in patients 65 years and older
- First trimester of pregnancy increases the risk of cardiovascular-related malformations such as atrial and/or ventricular septal defects in infants.
- Neonates exposed to sertraline late in the third trimester have been reported with complications requiring prolonged hospitalization, tube feeding, and respiratory support

## Pearls

- *Essential monitoring for unusual changes in behavior, anxiety, suicidality, or any other clinical signs of worsening illness.*
- *Regularly evaluate for depression and suicidality, especially when changing the dose of sertraline.*
- *Sertraline may also precipitate mania in patients at risk for bipolar disorder*
- *Safe in patients with a history of myocardial infarction, heart failure, and other cardiac conditions*
- *Safe in pregnancy and with breastfeeding*
- *The overdose of sertraline is generally well-tolerated*
- *Treatment of serotonin syndrome requires discontinuing the medication and supportive care*
- *It is important to note that antipyretics are likely not beneficial to patients experiencing hyperthermia due to serotonin syndrome.*

## Dosage Variations

Oral tablet form are 25mg, 50mg, 100mg, in capsules of 150mg, 200mg, and solution form 20mg/ml

Antidepressants

# Sertraline (Zoloft)

## Mechanism of Action

**Classification (SSSRI);** Sertraline is an antidepressant with primarily inhibitory effects on presynaptic serotonin reuptake. This inhibition of serotonin reuptake results in an accumulation of serotonin.

## Indications

- **Major depressive disorder (MDD)**
- **Obsessive-compulsive disorder (OCD)**
- **Social anxiety disorder (SAD)**
- **Panic disorder**
- **Posttraumatic stress disorder (PTSD)**
- **Generalized anxiety disorder (GAD)**
- **Premenstrual dysphoric disorder (PMDD)**
- **Vasomotor symptoms associated with menopause**
    - Not FDA approved for use in children and adolescents less than 18 years of age

**Off-Label Use:** OCD, SAD, BDD, PPD, Dysthymia

## Pharmacokinetics

- The steady-state mean value of T1/2 is 21 hours
- Undergoes metabolism via hepatic CYPP450 2D6
- Excretion is mainly via urine
- Plasma concentrations can potentially double following dosage increases of 50%

## Adverse Effects/Contraindications

1. Side effects are dose-dependent
2. The most common side effects include drowsiness, dry mouth, loss of appetite, sweating, sleep disturbance, and sexual side effects
3. Clinicians can address sexual side effects medications like sildenafil).
4. Discontinuation syndrome is more common and more severe with paroxetine than with other SSRIs
5. Withdrawal symptoms from discontinuation include dizziness, lethargy, nausea, vomiting, headache, fever, chills, vivid dreams, electric shock-like-sensation, dyskinesia, anxiety, crying, irritability, and depersonalization

## Pearls

- *Needs close observation and be monitored for worsening clinical symptoms, behavior changes (mania, social function, anxiety), or suicidal ideations*
- *Labs should include serum sodium concentration to rule out SIADH*
- *Vital signs should be monitored for signs of serotonergic hyperactivity*
- *Serotonin syndrome is treated by discontinuing any of the offending agents*
- *Rarely lethal in overdose by itself, patients can develop somnolence, nausea, tremor, heart rhythm disturbances, confusion, vomiting, dizziness, and mydriasis*
- *During toxicity, a patient's airway, oxygenation, and ventilation require evaluation first*
- *There is no specific treatment for paroxetine toxicity*

Antidepressants

# Desvenlafaxine (Pristiq)

## Dosage Variations

Starting dose is 50mg. 25mg (common choice for tapering off of the medication), 50mg, and 100mg tablet available only as an extended-release formulation. Max dose is 400mg.

## Mechanism of Action

**Classification (SNRIs);** Antidepressant medication belongs to a category of drugs that inhibits the reuptake of both serotonin and norepinephrine, known as SNRIs. Primary active metabolite of venlafaxine. In vitro studies have shown that Desvenlafaxine is ten times more selective for serotonin than for norepinephrine, making it similar to the drug duloxetine. It has an affinity to serotonin 30-times more than it does to norepinephrine.

## Indications

- **MDD**

**Off-label** to treat hot flashes during menopause

## Pharmacokinetics

- Half-life: 11 hours
- Metabolizes through the liver with a small amount broken down via the cytochrome P450 system
- Renal excretion is a major route of elimination

## Adverse Effects/Contraindications

1. It is important to consider treating with a lower dose when dealing with patients who have moderate to severe renal impairment or end-stage renal disease
2. Most common side effects are abdominal pain, decreased appetite, headache, and nausea
3. Less commonly noted were diarrhea, dizziness, and cough
4. Abruptly stopping the use of desvenlafaxine can cause irritability, nausea, and headaches
5. Gradually tapering the medication is recommended to avoid such side effects

## Pearls

- *A detailed assessment of depression and suicidality should take place, especially at the beginning of therapy or when the dosage is changed*
- *It is necessary to observe patients taking desvenlafaxine for behavior changes such as anxiety, social function, and mania*
- *Desvenlafaxine is rarely lethal when used as a standalone agent*
- *There is a risk of serotonin syndrome when combined with other serotonin augmenting medications, triptans, tricyclic antidepressants, over-the-counter agents, and monoamine oxidase inhibitors*
- *The treatment for overdose is symptomatic and supportive*
- *There is no specific treatment for desvenlafaxine toxicity*

Antidepressants

# Duloxetine (Cymbalta)

## Dosage Variations

Oral route with or without food intake (20mg, 30mg, 60mg). Should not be crushed or chewed. Can also be sprinkled on apple juice or apple sauce stable for 2 hours.

## Mechanism of Action

**Classification (SSNRIs):** Duloxetine is a serotonin-norepinephrine reuptake inhibitor (SNRI) that increases the levels of serotonin and norepinephrine in the brain by inhibiting their reuptake. Serotonin is involved in mood regulation, anxiety, and sleep, while norepinephrine affects alertness, arousal, and pain perception. By enhancing the availability of these neurotransmitters in the synaptic cleft, duloxetine improves mood, reduces anxiety, and can alleviate pain.

## Indications

- **Major depressive disorder**
- **Generalized anxiety disorder**
- **Fibromyalgia**
- **Chronic musculoskeletal pain**
- **Diabetic peripheral neuropathy**

**Off-label:** *chemotherapy-induced peripheral neuropathy and stress urinary incontinence in both men and women*

## Pharmacokinetics

- Half-life : 11 hours
- It metabolizes through the liver with a small amount broken down via the cytochrome P450 system
- Renal excretion is a major route of elimination
- Nearly 45% of the medication is unchanged when eliminated in the urine

## Adverse Effects/Contraindications

1. Headaches and drowsiness, and fatigue, are common
2. Excreted in breast milk and may produce effects in the nursing infant
3. Avoided in patients with liver failure or severe renal dysfunction as well as those patients receiving treatment with linezolid or intravenous methylene blue due to an increased risk of serotonin syndrome
4. Caution is necessary when prescribing duloxetine in the geriatric population

**Serious adverse effects of duloxetine include:**

- Suicidality
- Serotonin syndrome
- Hepatoxicity
- Mania
- Syncope
- Syndrome of inappropriate antidiuretic hormone secretion (SIADH)
- Hyponatremia

**Common adverse effects of duloxetine include:**

- Headache
- Drowsiness
- Fatigue
- Nausea
- Xerostomia
- Abdominal pain
- Weight loss
- Weakness
- Insomnia
- Dizziness
- Chane in libido
- Diaphoresis
- Constipation
- Decreased appetite
- Tremor
- Diarrhea
- Erectile dysfunction

## Pearls

- *Fatal outcomes have occurred with overdoses at as low as 1000 mg and there is no antidote to duloxetine overdose.*
- *Patients with abnormal vital signs need monitoring, and severe cases may warrant ICU-level of care*
- *check blood pressure and vitals before initiating therapy*
- *Patients should be monitored for abnormal bleeding as duloxetine may impair platelet aggregation*
- *Laboratory workup should include monitoring serum creatinine, blood urea nitrogen(BUN), transaminase levels, blood glucose levels, and HgbA1c in diabetic patients*
- *Electrolytes such as Sodium levels require follow-up when prescribing duloxetine in the geriatric population*

Antidepressants

# Venlafaxine (Effexor)

## Dosage Variations

Available in tablet and capsule. The oral tablets come in immediate-release (25mg, 37.5mg, 50mg, 75mg and 100mg) and extended-release forms (37.5mg, 75mg, 150mg, and 225mg.) The immediate-release tablet can be cut or crushed, but the extended-release tablet may not be.

## Mechanism of Action

**Classification (SNRIs):** Venlafaxine works by increasing serotonin levels, norepinephrine, and dopamine in the brain by blocking transport proteins and stopping their reuptake at the presynaptic terminal. This action leads to more transmitters available at the synapse and ultimately increases the stimulation of postsynaptic receptors.

## Indications

- **Depression**
- **Social anxiety disorder**
- **Cataplexy**

**Off-label:** attention deficit disorder, fibromyalgia, diabetic neuropathy, complex pain syndromes, hot flashes, migraine prevention, post-traumatic stress disorder, obsessive-compulsive disorder, and premenstrual dysphoric disorder

## Pharmacokinetics

- Half-life: Approximately 11 hours.
- Metabolism: Venlafaxine is primarily metabolized in the liver, with a small amount broken down via the cytochrome P450 system. This system includes enzymes such as CYP2D6 and CYP3A4, which play a role in the metabolism of many drugs.
- Excretion: Renal excretion is a major route of Desvenlafaxine elimination, which is the active metabolite of venlafaxine

## Adverse Effects/Contraindications

- Venlafaxine causes a lower frequency of anticholinergic, sedating, and cardiovascular side effects but a higher incidence of gastrointestinal complaints, sleep impairment, and sexual dysfunction than TCAs
- Impair sexual function, resulting in diminished libido, impotence, or difficulty achieving orgasm
- Some patients find withdrawal symptoms uncomfortable.
- Can also cause abnormal bleeding, altered platelet function, and anaphylaxis/anaphylactoid reaction
- Can cause fatal skin conditions such as Stevens-Johnson syndrome, toxic epidermal necrolysis, and erythema multiforme
- Increase risk of serotonin syndrome, thought to result from hyperstimulation of brainstem 5HT-1A receptors

**Common side effects include:**

- Headache
- Nausea
- Insomnia, dizziness, hypotension, anorexia, somnolence
- Xerostomia
- Asthenia
- HTN
- Impotence, decreased libido, and/or anorgasmia
- Constipation
- Weight loss
- Abnormal dreams
- Diarrhea, abdominal pain
- Blurred vision
- Anxiety, tremor
- Hypercholesterolemia
- Hyponatremia
- Serotonin syndrome[6]
- Seizures

## Pearls

- *Patients should not take venlafaxine with monoamine oxidase inhibitors (MAOIs), linezolid, and methylene blue*
- *For >18yrs old. It should be taken with food, and patients should not take it with alcohol as combining alcohol and venlafaxine can lead to increased sedation*
- *Should not be combined with drugs for weight loss, such as phentermine*
- *Venlafaxine with cimetidine raises the risk of high blood pressure or liver disease*
- *Venlafaxine with haloperidol raises the risk of QT prolongation*
- *Venlafaxine taken with warfarin and anti-inflammatory drugs such as aspirin, ibuprofen, naproxen (NSAIDs) increase the risk of bleeding*
- *Ritonavir, clarithromycin, or ketoconazole can inhibit the breakdown of venlafaxine leading to venlafaxine accumulation in the body*
- *Venlafaxine, taken with zolpidem, lorazepam, and diphenhydramine, can lead to increased sedation.*
- *Metoprolol may be less effective when taken with venlafaxine*
- *Venlafaxine can cause false positives when testing the patient's urine for phencyclidine (PCP) and amphetamine. This effect may remain for several days after stopping venlafaxine*
- *Symptoms of an overdose of venlafaxine can include: tachycardia, unusual sleepiness, dilated pupils, seizures, vomiting, cardiac arrhythmias, hypotension, muscle aches or pains, or dizziness*
- *Hunter Toxicity Criteria Decision Rules can be used to form the diagnosis*

Antidepressants

# Mirtazapine (Remeron)

## Dosage Variations

Start 15mg/day which patients can take without regard to meals, administered as a single dose of an oral tablet. The most effective range is around 15mg to 45mg daily.

## Mechanism of Action

**Classification (SNRIs);** It inhibits the central presynaptic alpha-2-adrenergic receptors, which causes an increased release of serotonin and norepinephrine. Mirtazapine is also sometimes called a noradrenergic and specific serotonergic antidepressant (NaSSA)

## Indications

**FDA-approved**

- **Major depressive disorders**

## Pharmacokinetics

- Rapidly absorbed, and peak plasma concentrations are attained in 2 hours
- Half-life: 20 to 40 hours
- Metabolites of mirtazapine are excreted primarily via urine
- Metabolized in the liver and cytochrome P450 enzymes (CYP1A2, CYP2D6, and CYP3A4)

## Adverse Effects/Contraindications

- Drowsiness
- Weight gain
- Xerostomia
- Increased serum cholesterol
- Constipation
- Increase in appetite
- Sedation
- Thrombocytopenia
- Bone marrow suppression and neutropenia
- Hypertriglyceridemia
- Acute pancreatitis (rare but life-threatening ADR)
- Transient alterations of liver function tests and rare cases of acute liver injury
- Caution is advised in patients with cardiovascular disorders
- Lipid profile with weight gain

## Pearls

- *Agranulocytosis or severe neutropenia (such as stomatitis, sore throat, other possible signs of infection, or a low WBC)*
- *Clinicians should monitor renal and liver function and the drug levels in the blood of elderly patients because clearance is reduced*
- *Taking mirtazapine with other sedative drugs can severely increase the sedative effect*
- *In the event of an overdose, mirtazapine is a relatively safe drug*
- *Signs and symptoms associated with overdose also were associated with disorientation, drowsiness, and impaired memory*
- *It is important to note that there are no specific antidotes for mirtazapine*

Antidepressants

# Trazodone (Desyrel)

## Dosage Variations

Orally available in tablets 50mg, 100mg, 150mg, and 300mg in the US. Up to 600mg per day in hospitalized patients and 100mg per day for elderly.

## Mechanism of Action

**Classification (Serotonin antagonist and reuptake inhibitor):** Trazodone is an antidepressant that works by inhibiting both serotonin transporter and serotonin type 2 receptors (serotonin antagonism and serotonin reuptake inhibiting effects). It is a triazolopyridine derivative. Trazodone inhibits the reuptake of serotonin and blocks the histamine and alpha-1-adrenergic receptors.

## Indications

- **Major depressive disorders**

**Non-FDA-approved Uses**

- Patients with sleep problems
- Anxiety
- Alzheimer disease
- Substance abuse
- Bulimia
- Fibromyalgia
- Post-traumatic stress disorder (PTSD)

## Pharmacokinetics

- Half-life: 7-10 hr
- Excretion: Urine
- Dialyzable: No
- Metabolism: hepatic P450 enzyme CYP3A4 (major) CYP2D6 (minor)

## Adverse Effects/Contraindications

- The primary adverse effects of trazodone include headaches, fatigue, dizziness, and drowsiness/somnolence
- Other risks include anticholinergic effects (dry mouth), orthostatic hypotension, QT prolongation, torsades, priapism, and an increase in suicidal thoughts
- It increased risk of suicidal thinking, especially in younger adults, adolescents, and children
- Special care is necessary for men that have disease processes that will affect the penis or vascularization as it can cause priapism
- Baseline liver functions require monitoring
- Monitor also for signs or symptoms of serotonin syndrome and cardiovascular adverse effects

## Pearls

- *Patients receiving trazodone should also be monitored for suicide ideation, especially at the beginning of the treatment or when the dose is modified*
- *Health care providers should assess the response to trazodone therapy and consider augmenting or switching antidepressants if inadequate response*
- *Special care is necessary for patients with severe hepatic impairment and severe renal impairment.*
- *Overdose can precipitate arrhythmias, respiratory arrest, coma, and priapism*
- *If priapism occurs, it requires urgent urologist intervention*
- *The medical team should call the local poison center for up-to-date guidance on trazodone overdose*

Antidepressants

# Vilazodone (Viibryd)

## Dosage Variations

10-mg, 20mg, and 40mg (recommended dosage). Titrated starting with an initial dosage of 10mg once daily for 7 days, followed by 20mg, and then to 40mg once daily.

## Mechanism of Action

**Classification (SSRIs):** The mechanism of the antidepressant effect of vilazodone is thought to be related to its enhancement of serotonergic activity in the CNS through selective inhibition of serotonin reuptake. Vilazodone binds with high affinity to the serotonin reuptake site but not to the norepinephrine or dopamine reuptake site. As a result, vilazodone potently and selectively inhibits the reuptake of serotonin.

## Indications

- **Major depressive disorders**

## Pharmacokinetics

- Pharmacokinetic activity (5–80 mg) is dose-proportional
- Terminal half-life is approximately 25 hours
- Metabolized in the liver, primarily via the cytochrome P450 (CYP) 3A4 isoenzyme

## Adverse Effects/Contraindications

**BOXED WARNING**

- Increased the risk of suicidal thinking and behavior in adolescents, and young adults
- Not approved for use in pediatric patients
- Should be taken with food
- Main SE: diarrhea, nausea, insomnia, and vomiting
- Other adverse effects included dizziness, dry mouth, fatigue, abnormal dreams, decreased libido, arthralgia, and palpitations
- Vilazodone should be taken with food

## Pearls

- *Should be monitored for clinical worsening and for suicidal thinking or behavior, especially during the initial few months and at times of dose increases or decreases*
- *Associated with symptoms upon discontinuation, including dysphoric mood, irritability, agitation, anxiety, and confusion*
- *The most severe form of serotonin syndrome resembles NMS and is characterized by hyperthermia, muscle rigidity, autonomic instability with possible rapid fluctuation of vital signs, and alterations in mental status*
- *Patients receiving warfarin therapy should be carefully monitored*

Antidepressants

# Vortioxetine (Trintellix)

## Dosage Variations

- Starting dose of 10mg a day and can be increased to 20mg and decrease to 5mg a day
- Can be discontinued abruptly

## Mechanism of Action

**Classification (SSRIs):** This is an antidepressant medication that works by blocking the serotonin transporter (SERT) and acting as a partial agonist at serotonin 5-HT1A receptors.

## Indications

- **Major depressive disorders**

## Pharmacokinetics

- Half-life: approx. 66 hours
- Absorbed in the gastrointestinal tract and exhibits peak plasma concentrations in about seven to 11 hours
- Consumption of food does not affect the bioavailability
- Metabolized primarily through oxidation via CYP2D6, CYP3A4/5, CYP2C19, CYP2C9, CYP2A6, CYP2C8, and CYP2B6 and subsequent glucuronic acid conjugation
- Primarily eliminated in urine

## Adverse Effects/Contraindications

- The most common adverse drug events were nausea, headache, dry mouth, and dizziness.
- Serious adverse effects that occurred were hypertensive crisis, increased risk of suicide, and pancreatitis
- The incidence of sexual adverse effects is evident for both men and women

## Pearls

- *Safe for Pregnancy and Breastfeeding*
- *Weight neutral*

Antidepressants

# Bupropion (Wellbutrin)

## Dosage Variations

Immediate-Release (IR) Tablets:

- 75 mg
- 100 mg

Extended-Release (XL) Tablets:

- 150 mg

## Mechanism of Action

**Classification (un-classified) :** It's an antidepressant with a mechanism that is not fully understood. Bupropion seems not to affect monoamine uptake but is known to inhibit the reuptake of norepinephrine and dopamine weakly. The effects on norepinephrine and dopamine appear to lead to its clinical manifestations. Dopamine reuptake inhibition is reportedly very high, while norepinephrine uptake is less potent. Bupropion also acts to a lesser degree on nicotinic and serotonin receptors.

## Indications

- **MDD**
- **Seasonal affective disorder**
- **Smoking cessation**

**Off-label:** antidepressant-induced sexual dysfunction, attention-deficit/hyperactivity disorder (ADHD), depression associated with bipolar disorder, and obesity

In the pediatric population, bupropion is used off-label for ADHD

## Pharmacokinetics

- Metabolized in the liver by CYP2B6
- Drug's elimination is primarily in the urine
- The half-life is 3 to 4 hours distribution, but the half-life extends to about 21 hours when dosed chronically

## Adverse Effects/Contraindications

- Main SE:
- Cardiovascular (tachycardia)
- Respiratory (rhinitis, pharyngitis)
- Central nervous system (insomnia, headache, agitation, dizziness)
- Dermatologic (diaphoresis)
- Endocrine (weight loss)
- Gastrointestinal (constipation, dry mouth, nausea)
- Musculoskeletal (tremor)
- Ophthalmologic (blurred vision)

## Pearls

- *Does not require monitoring with serum testing*
- *There are no firmly established therapeutic concentrations of the drug*
- *Before prescribing, the provider should determine if any existing medications interact with bupropion. Common interactions include many antidepressants, clopidogrel, and other drugs that lower the seizure threshold*
- *Patients need to limit alcohol intake while on bupropion*
- *Requires caution in breastfeeding individuals because the drug and its metabolites are secreted into breast milk.*
- *Other effects include hallucinations, mental status changes, agitation, arrhythmias.*
- *Bupropion abuse is rare, but reports do exist*
- *The most severe adverse effects are lowered seizure threshold and the potential of worsening suicidal ideation.*

Antidepressants

# Amitriptyline (Elavil)

## Dosage Variations

Oral tablets of 10mg, 25mg, 50mg, 75mg, 100mg, and 150mg. Administer amitriptyline at night time, as it can lead to sedation

## Mechanism of Action

**Classification (un-classified) :** It's an antidepressant with a mechanism that is not fully understood. Bupropion seems not to affect monoamine uptake but is known to inhibit the reuptake of norepinephrine and dopamine weakly. The effects on norepinephrine and dopamine appear to lead to its clinical manifestations. Dopamine reuptake inhibition is reportedly very high, while norepinephrine uptake is less potent. Bupropion also acts to a lesser degree on nicotinic and serotonin receptors.

## Indications

- **Major Depressive Disorder**

**Non-FDA-approved:** anxiety, post-traumatic stress disorder, insomnia, chronic pain (diabetic neuropathy, fibromyalgia), irritable bowel syndrome, interstitial cystitis (bladder pain syndrome), migraine prophylaxis, postherpetic neuralgia, and sialorrhea

Amitriptyline has been used for post-COVID headaches

## Pharmacokinetics

- Well absorbed following oral administration
- The bioavailability is high first-pass metabolism.
- Metabolized to nortriptyline by CYP2C19, CYP3A4 and CYP2D6
- Half-life: 10 to 28 hours
- Its metabolites are primarily excreted by the kidney

## Adverse Effects/Contraindications

- Most commonly SE: weight gain and gastrointestinal symptoms like constipation, xerostomia, dizziness, headache, and somnolence
- The drug can increase the risk of suicidal ideation and behavior in adolescents and young adults
- Due to its alpha-adrenergic receptor blockade, can cause orthostatic hypotension, dizziness, and sedation.
- Can also cause heart rate variability, slow intracardiac conduction, induce various arrhythmias, and cause QTc (corrected QT) prolongation - CAUTION FOR CARDIAC
- Anticholinergic side effects include blurred vision, dry mouth, urinary retention, tachycardia, acute angle glaucoma, confusion, and delirium
- Antihistamine side effects secondary to its histamine (H1) receptor binding property include sedation, increased appetite, weight gain, confusion, and delirium
- Amitriptyline can decrease the seizure threshold
- It can increase the risk of bone fracture and (rare) bone marrow suppression

## Pearls

- *Body Mass Index, liver function test, thyroid function test, and serum amitriptyline concentrations requires monitoring*
- *should monitor for increased suicidality and unusual behavior changes, especially during the first 1 to 2 months*
- *Administer amitriptyline at night time, as it can lead to sedation*
- *Amitriptyline toxicity can be serious and even fatal, which may require admission to the ICU for monitoring*
- *Seizures secondary to overdose are treatable with diazepam or lorazepam*
- *Intravenous lipid emulsion (ILE) has been used in severe overdose*
- *Amitriptyline can cross the placental barrier*

Antidepressants

# Amoxapine (Asendin)

## Dosage Variations

Oral tablet formulations, with strengths of 25mg, 50mg, 100mg, and 150mg doses.

## Mechanism of Action

**Classification (tricyclic antidepressant (TCA):** Amoxapine, a second-generation tricyclic dibenzoxazepine antidepressant, primarily functions by inhibiting the reuptake of norepinephrine in neuronal synapses. The drug exhibits minimal effect on the histamine H1 receptor and serotonin receptors, except for the serotonin-6 receptor (HTR-6, 5-HT-6). Amoxapine also acts as a dopamine (DA) receptor antagonist, specifically targeting D2 and D4 receptors.

## Indications

**FDA-Approved Indications**

- **Treatment-resistant depression:**
  - in cases of depression accompanied by other psychiatric issues such as anxiety, agitation, psychosis, neurosis, or recurrent depression

**Off-Label Uses**

Reduce the incidence of diarrhea in patients undergoing chemotherapy, particularly when used in conjunction with irinotecan

## Pharmacokinetics

- Rapidly absorbed in the body after oral administration
- Plasma concentration for approx 90 minutes
- Undergoes hepatic metabolism primarily via the CYP2D6 enzyme
- The active metabolite, 8-hydroxy-amoxapine, has a half-life of 30 hours, whereas the drug has a half-life of 8 hours
- Primary route of drug elimination is through urine

## Adverse Effects/Contraindications

- Insomnia, palpitations, tachycardia, hypotension, and constipation common effects
- May trigger hypomanic states in individuals with underlying bipolar disorder
- Associated with instances of painful ejaculations relieved by the administration of tamsulosin
- Amoxapine's anticholinergic properties can result in adverse effects such as sedation, dry mouth, delirium, and drug-induced Parkinsonism, particularly among older patients
- Use of the drug with barbiturates and alcohol should be avoided

## Pearls

- *Should undergo regular monitoring for resolution or reduction of symptoms, withdrawal symptoms from abrupt discontinuation, changes in body weight and BMI, blood pressure and blood glucose levels*
- *Older individuals and those with preexisting cardiac disease or hyperthyroidism should undergo a 12-lead electrocardiogram as part of their evaluation*
- *Electrolyte monitoring in patients 65 and older is important*
- *The primary concern for TCA toxicity is the potential development of serotonin syndrome, particularly when the medication is combined with other antidepressants such as SSRIs or SNRIs*

Antidepressants

# Clomipramine (Anafranil)

## Dosage Variations

Capsule form as a hydrochloride salt, with dosages of 25mg, 50mg, and 75mg.
The max dose for both children and adults is 250mg/day.

## Mechanism of Action

**Classification (TCA):** Clomipramine is a serotonin reuptake inhibitor (S-RI) with a stronger affinity for the serotonin transporter (SERT) than other TCAs and S-RIs. The resulting action of clomipramine increases serotonergic and noradrenergic transmission.

## Indications

**FDA-Approved Indication**

- Obsessive-compulsive disorder (OCD)
  - in ages ten and older

**Off-Label Uses**

Off-label conditions:

- Depression
- Anxiety
- Treatment-resistant depression
- Cataplexy syndrome
- Insomnia
- Neuropathic pain
- Chronic pain
- Body dysmorphic disorder
- Panic disorder
- Premature ejaculation
- Pediatric nocturnal enuresis
- Trichotillomania

## Pharmacokinetics

- Metabolism of clomipramine is primarily through the liver via oxidation by CYP450 2D6.
- The half-life of clomipramine is 17 to 28 hours

## Adverse Effects/Contraindications

- The adverse effects of clomipramine include nausea, weight gain, increased appetite, sedation, dry mouth, constipation, urinary retention, blurred vision, headache, dizziness, fatigue, hypotension, anxiety, restlessness, sweating, blue-green urine, and sexual dysfunction
- Life-threatening adverse effects include arrhythmia, tachycardia, QTc prolongation, orthostasis, seizures, paralytic ileus, hyperthermia, hepatic failure, increased intraocular pressure, mania induction, and activation of suicidality
- Adverse effects of clomipramine have been found in fetuses, as the medication crosses the placenta

## Pearls

- *Electrocardiogram (EKG) testing is a recommendation at baseline and after reaching therapeutic effect*
- *Weight, body mass index (BMI), fasting plasma glucose, and fasting lipids are recommended at baseline and during treatment*
- *Toxicity with doses over 300 mg per day*
- *The most common symptoms seen in toxicity are arrhythmias, seizures, and hypotension*
- *Coma and death may also occur in severe overdoses*
- *The antidote in serotonin syndrome is cyproheptadine, along with supportive care of vital signs*

Antidepressants

# Desipramine (Norpramin )

## Dosage Variations

Orally and comes in tablets of 10mg, 25mg, 50mg, 75mg, 100mg, and 150mg. Max dose is 300mg a day.

## Mechanism of Action

**Classification (TCA):** It blocks the reuptake of norepinephrine and serotonin in the presynaptic neuronal membrane. It also proposed to have alpha-1 blocking, antihistamine, and anticholinergic effects as well.

## Indications

**FDA-Approved Indication**

- Depression

**Off-label use:** bulimia nervosa, irritable bowel syndrome, neuropathic pain, overactive bladder, postherpetic neuralgia, and ADHD.

*Desipramine has shown mild effectiveness in the treatment of ADHD.*

## Pharmacokinetics

- Half-Life elimination: 15-24hr
- Onset: 2-5 days (initial therapeutic effect); 2-3 wk (full effect)
- Peak Plasma Time: 4-6 hr
- Excretion: Urine
- Metabolism: Hepatic CYP2D6
- First Pass : Liver

## Adverse Effects/Contraindications

- Increased risk for suicide, orthostatic hypotension, cardiac abnormalities, seizures, ocular crisis, and fractures
- Orthostatic hypotension, likely due to blockade of alpha one receptors, is a common reason for discontinuation of this drug
- Knowing the history of cardiac disease within the family is a strong recommendation before the prescription
- Patients with a family history of sudden death, cardiac dysrhythmia, or cardiac conduction distances should have close monitoring

## Pearls

- *Treatment with this drug requires a minimum of 2 to 3 weeks to see the full effect*
- *Extreme precautions should be taken in patients with cardiovascular disease*
- *resulted in a higher death rate compared to other tricyclic antidepressants*
- *Gastrointestinal decontamination should be initiated via activated charcoal as soon as possible*
- *Emesis is contraindicated*
- *Increased risk of suicide in ages 24 and younger is one of the most significant*

Antidepressants

# Doxepin (Silenor & Sinequan)

## Dosage Variations

- Oral tablets 3mg, and 6mg
- Oral capsules 10mg, 25mg, 50mg, 75mg, 100mg, & 150mg.
- Oral solutions as 10mg/mL.
- Topical creams (5%) and transdermal patches.

## Mechanism of Action

**Classification (TCA):** Depression appears to result from a chemical imbalance and a lack of neurotransmitters in the brain. The different classes of antidepressant medications have been formulated to perform unique mechanisms by targeting different receptors and increasing the availability of neurotransmitters. Doxepin is in the tricyclic antidepressants (TCA) drug class; these agents work by increasing the concentration of the neurotransmitter's serotonin (5-HT) and norepinephrine (NE) in the brain.

## Indications

- **Major depressive disorder**
- **Insomnia**
- **Skin pruritus**

**Off-label:** Neuropathic Pain, Migraines, Urethral Irritation and Dysuria

## Pharmacokinetics

**Pharmacokinetics for Oral Formulation**
Peak plasma concentration: 3.5 hours
Metabolism: Hepatic; active metabolite is desmethyldoxepin
Half-life: approximately 15 hours to 31 hours

**Pharmacokinetics for Topical Formulation**
Absorption: Percutaneous absorption
Metabolism: Hepatic;
Half-life elimination: Doxepin: 28 to 52 hours for desmethyldoxepin

## Adverse Effects/Contraindications

- Antagonizes three different receptors, which include: histamine, adrenergic, and muscarinic
- Proper education is necessary to prevent patients from self-medicating and overdosing on such pills
- Has the potential to cause a significant increase in weight
- Carefully monitored in those with cardiovascular disorders because it can cause orthostatic hypotension
- Cause neurological effects such as coma, grand mal seizures, and respiratory depression

## Pearls

- *Side effects occurred more often when the serum levels were above the therapeutic range*
- *One of the most frequently ingested used for self-poison in an attempt to commit suicide*
- *Overdose on doxepin can affect the central nervous system and cardiovascular system*
- *Doxepin is known to block sodium and potassium channels on cardiomyocytes*
- *Cause neurological effects such as coma, grand mal seizures, and respiratory depression*
- *Treatment includes sodium bicarbonate, hemodialysis/hemoperfusion, and supportive therapy*

Antidepressants

# Imipramine (Tofranil)

## Dosage Variations

The tablets are available in doses of 10mg, 25mg, 50mg, while the capsules are available in doses of 75mg, 100mg, 125mg, 150mg.

## Mechanism of Action

**Classification (TCA):** Imipramine blocks the reuptake of norepinephrine and serotonin. Since imipramine is a tertiary amine, it has a greater affinity for serotonin, and it has more anticholinergic side effects, which can prove helpful in treating enuresis. Imipramine blocks D-2 receptors.

## Indications

- **Depression**

**Off label use:** Chronic Neuropathic Pain and Panic Disorder; adjunctive therapy in nocturnal enuresis in children above six years of age

## Pharmacokinetics

- Completely Absorbed
- Peak plasma time: 1-2 hr
- Hepatic CYP1A2, CYP2C19, CYP2D6
- Half-life: 6-18 hr
- Excretion: Urine

## Adverse Effects/Contraindications

- Antihistaminic effects of imipramine can lead to dizziness, sedation, confusion, delirium, seizures, increased appetite, and weight gain
- Cardiac arrhythmia, which is the leading cause of death in tricyclic antidepressant overdose
- Other adverse effects include GI upset, mild elevation of liver enzymes, sexual dysfunction, and diaphoresis

## Pearls

- *Regular drug monitoring is required to ensure the therapeutic blood level*
- *Treatment requires a duration of around 4 to 5 weeks to elicit a good response*
- *Extreme precautions are necessary, especially in a patient with cardiovascular disease*
- *An overdose of imipramine can result in serious side effects, mainly cardiac dysrhythmia, critical hypotension, convulsions, coma, confusion, hyperactive reflexes, and hypothermia*

Antidepressants

# Nortriptyline

(Pamelor & Aventyl HCL)

## Dosage Variations

Capsule form comes in 10 mg, 25 mg, 50 mg, and 75 mg strengths. The oral solution is 10 mg/5 mL (473 mL). >150 mg daily is not recommended.

## Mechanism of Action

**Classification (TCA):** The consensus is that Nortriptyline inhibits the reuptake of serotonin and norepinephrine by the presynaptic neuronal membrane, thereby increasing the concentration of those neurotransmitters in the synapse. It also inhibits the activity of histamine, 5-hydroxytryptamine, and acetylcholine.

## Indications

**Depression**

- is not FDA approved for use in children.

**Off-label indications:**

- Chronic pain
- Diabetic neuropathy
- Persistent myofascial pain
- Trigeminal neuralgia
- Postherpetic neuralgia
- Smoking cessation
- Migraine prophylaxis
- Neurogenic cough

## Pharmacokinetics

- Peak plasma concentrations are 7 to 8.5 hours
- It is distributed to the brain, heart, and liver
- Undergoes first-pass metabolism in the liver by CYP2D6
- Excreted in urine but it is also excreted in feces via the bile

## Adverse Effects/Contraindications

- Increased risk of suicide in adolescents, children, and young adults
- The most common adverse effects of nortriptyline includes:

1. Downiness
2. *Xerostomia*
3. *Dizziness*
4. Constipation
5. Blurred visions
6. Palpitations
7. *Tachycardia*
8. Impaired coordination
9. Increased appetite
10. *Nausea/vomiting*
11. *Diaphoresis*
12. Weakness
13. Disorientation
14. Confusion
15. Restlessness
16. Insomnia
17. Anxiety/agitation
18. *Urinary retention*
19. Urinary frequency
20. Rash
21. Urticaria
22. Pruritus
23. *Weight gain*
24. Libido changes
25. Impotence
26. Gynecomastia
27. Galactorrhea
28. Tremor
29. Hypo/hyperglycemia
30. Paresthesia
31. Photosensitivity

- The **most serious adverse effects include:** orthostatic hypotension, HTN, syncope, ventricular arrhythmias, AV block, MI, stroke, paralytic ileus, glaucoma, increased IOP, agranulocytosis, leukopenia, thrombocytopenia, hepatitis, angioedema
- Neuropsychiatric adverse drug reactions include EPS symptoms, ataxia, tardive dyskinesia, hallucinations, psychosis exacerbation, hypomania/mania, exacerbation of depression, suicidality, serotonin syndrome, SIADH, hyperthermia, and seizures

## Pearls

- *This med crosses the placenta, and is present in breast milk*
- *Clinicians should frequently monitor cardiac parameters*
- *Monitor for improvement/worsening of depression using questionnaires such as PHQ-9 and the Montgomery-Asberg Depression Rating Scale (MADRS)*
- *Toxicity can be very harmful to the body. The most crucial initial step when assessing a patient with toxicity is ensuring the patient can adequately breathe*
- *It is recommended that the clinician contact the local poison control center for specific pediatric treatment*

Antidepressants

# Protriptyline (Vivactil)

## Dosage Variations

- Available in tablets of 5 mg or 10mg.
- Initiate at 15mg to 40mg a day
- Divide the dose into 3 or 4 doses, not to be taken all at one time
- Max dose 60mg

## Mechanism of Action

**Classification (TCA):** These often decrease in people who are depressed and are the main targets of antidepressants. Protriptyline has the fastest onset of action among other tricyclic antidepressants, and thus clinical effects can occur within the first week of use.

## Indications

**FDA-Approved Uses**

- Mental depression
- Narcolepsy
- Attention deficit hyperactivity disorder
- Headaches

**Non-FDA-Approved Uses**

- Treatment-resistant depression
- Local anesthetic
- Smoking cessation
- Cocaine dependence
- Apnea

## Pharmacokinetics

- Half-Life: 54-92 hr
- Peak Plasma Time: 24-30 hr
- Bioavailability: Completely absorbed
- Metabolism: Hepatic
- Excretion: Urine

## Adverse Effects/Contraindications

Among the TCAs, protriptyline is the most likely to cause tachycardia, hypotension, anxiety, and agitation, and for this reason, some European countries have discontinued protriptyline use

**Adverse Effects (like all TCAs)**

- CNS depression
- Convulsions
- Cardiac toxicity
- Weight gain
- Coma

**Rare, More Serious Adverse Effects**

- Hepatic failure
- Increased intraocular pressure
- Induction of mania
- Paralytic ileus
- Extrapyramidal symptoms
- QTc prolongation, arrhythmia, tachycardia, myocardial infarction
- Stroke, seizures, coma
- Sudden death

**Most Common Adverse Effects**

- Anxiety
- Agitation
- Apathy
- Anorexia
- Nausea
- Headache
- Diarrhea
- Constipation
- Urinary retention
- Dizziness
- Restlessness
- Insomnia (decrease of REM sleep)
- Nightmares
- Hypotension
- Hyponatremia
- Diaphoresis
- Itching
- Rash
- Blurred vision
- Dry mouth Impotence
- Change of libido
- Impotence
- Difficulty having an orgasm
- Suicidal thoughts and suicide attempts (black box warning) and risk, especially in that younger than 24 years old, is greater during the initial two months of starting the drug and during dosage adjustment

## Pearls

- *Taking more than recommended or taking the daily dose at one time can have significant consequences which can manifest in cardiac arrhythmias or EKG changes, especially QRS-widening hypotension, confusion, visual hallucinations, delusions, ataxia, tremors, syndrome of inappropriate ADH, tinnitus, hyperactive reflexes, muscle rigidity stupor, convulsions, coma, and even death*
- *ECG is a recommendation and close monitoring for patients over the age of 50, especially in those taking more than 20 mg per day, due to sensitivity to anticholinergic, cardiovascular, hypotensive, and sedative effects*
- *It is not recommended in patients under the age of 12 or intended for those under the age of 6*
- *It is a very potent TCA and a dangerous drug for overdose*

## Dosage Variations

Capsule

- 25mg
- 50mg
- 100mg

Antidepressants

# Trimipramine (Surmontil)

## Mechanism of Action

**Classification (TCA):** Neurotransmitter (esp NE & serotonin) reuptake inhibitor; inhibits reuptake by neuronal membrane; may also downregulate beta-adrenergic receptors and serotonin receptors.

## Indications

- **Major depressive disorder (MDD)**

## Pharmacokinetics

- Half-Life elimination: 16-40 hr
- Peak Plasma Time: 2 hr
- Metabolism: Hepatic
- Excretion: Urine

## Adverse Effects/Contraindications

**Frequency Not Defined**

- Sedation (less than amitriptyline, but greater than imipramine)
- Fatigue
- Dry mouth
- Constipation
- Blurred vision
- Weakness
- Lethargy
- Headache
- Agitation
- Insomnia
- Nausea/vomiting
- Anxiety
- Sweating
- Confusion
- EPS
- Dizziness
- Tinnitus
- Paresthesia
- Orthostatic hypotension
- ECG changes
- Tachycardia
- Incr LFTs
- Sexual dysfunction
- Rash
- Seizure (rare)
- Agranulocytosis, thrombocytopenia, eosinophilia, leukopenia (rare)
- SIADH (rare)

**Black Box Warnings**

- Increased risk of suicidal in patient <24 years of age
- slight decrease in suicidal thinking was seen in adults >65 years
- Patients should be monitored closely for changes in behavior, clinical worsening, and suicidal tendencies; this should be done during initial 1-2 months of therapy and dosage adjustments
- The patient's family should communicate any abrupt changes in behavior to the healthcare provider

## Pearls

- *This drug is not approved for use in pediatric patients*

Section 2

# Mood Stabilizers

Mood Stabilizers

# Lithium

## Dosage Variations

The tablet is available 450mg. Capsules in 150mg, 300mg, and 600mg. The liquid formulation is available as 8mEq/ 5 mL strength. Usually starts at 300mg twice or three times a day.

## Mechanism of Action

**Classification (Antimanic Drug):** The mechanism of action of lithium is not known. It is rapidly absorbed, has a small volume of distribution, and is excreted in the urine unchanged (there is no metabolism of lithium).

Lithium modifies sodium transport in nerve and muscle cells. It alters the metabolism of neurotransmitters, specifically catecholamines and serotonin. It may alter intracellular signaling via second messenger systems by inhibition of inositol monophosphate.

## Indications

- **Manic episode in bipolar disorder**
- **Maintenance therapy of bipolar disorder in a patient with a history of a manic episode**

***Off Label Use:*** major depressive disorder as an adjunct therapy, bipolar disorder without a history of mania, treatment of vascular headaches, and neutropenia

## Pharmacokinetics

- Bioavailability: Absorption increased by food
- Peak plasma time: 4.5-8.4 hr
- Metabolized by hepatic cytochrome P450 enzymes
- Half-life: 26 hr
- Dialyzable: No
- Excretion: mostly feces

## Adverse Effects/Contraindications

Lithium can cause several adverse effects. Typically the side effects are dose-related. Notable side effects include:

- Cardiac: Bradycardia, flattened or inverted T waves, heart block, and sick sinus syndrome.
- CNS: Confusion, memory problems, new or worsening tremor, hyperreflexia, clonus, slurred speech, ataxia, stupor, delirium, coma, and seizures (rarely). These effects are theoretically due to excess action on the same sites that mediate therapeutic action
- Renal: Nephrogenic diabetes insipidus with polyuria and polydipsia. These side effects are due to lithium's action on ion transport
- Hematologic: Leukocytosis and aplastic anemia
- Gastroenterological: Diarrhea and nausea
- Endocrinal: Euthyroid goiter or hypothyroid goiter
- Other: Acne, rash, and weight gain.

## Pearls

- *Drug is excreted in breast milk; not recommended*
- *Kidney function tests and thyroid function tests are needed before starting treatment*
- *> 50 years of age, an electrocardiogram is also necessary*
- *It is also beneficial to determine if the patient has prediabetes, diabetes, or dyslipidemia*
- *Monitor patients for dehydration and lower the dose when there are signs of infection, excessive sweating, or diarrhea*
- *Toxic levels are when the drug level is more than 1.5 mEq/L.*
- *Lithium toxicity has no antidote*
- *Avoid all diuretics when in lithium*
- *Lithium-induced weight gain is more common in women than in men*

Mood Stabilizers

# Valproate (Depakote/Valproic Acid)

## Dosage Variations

- Tablet in delayed release(125mg,250mg,500mg)
- Tablet in extended release (250mg & 500mg)
- Capsule (125mg)
- IV concentration (100mg/ml)

## Mechanism of Action

**Classification (Anticonvulsants):** May increase levels of the inhibitory neurotransmitter gamma-aminobutyric acid (GABA) in brain; may enhance or mimic action of GABA at postsynaptic receptor sites; may also inhibit sodium and calcium channels.

## Indications

- **Absence seizures**
- **Migraine Prophylaxes'**

***Off-Label Uses***

- *Manic episodes associated with bipolar disorder*
- *Emergency treatment of status epilepticus*
- *Diabetic peripheral neuropathy*
- *Post-herpetic neuralgia*
- *Impulsivity, agitation, and aggression*

## Pharmacokinetics

- Half-life: 7-13 hr (>2 months); 9-16 hr (adults)
- Peak plasma time: 2 hr
- Peak plasma concentration: 115-145 mcg/mL (IV)
- Metabolized by liver
- Enzymes inhibited: CYP2C9
- Excretion: Urine

## Adverse Effects/Contraindications

**Common Adverse Effects of VPA**

- The common adverse effects of VPA include gastrointestinal, neurological, and hematological symptoms
- The adverse effects associated with the medication include headache, abdominal pain, somnolence, dizziness, thrombocytopenia, asthenia, nausea and vomiting, diarrhea, tremor, weight changes, alopecia, constipation, emotional lability, insomnia, petechiae and ecchymosis, depression, rash, nervousness, appetite changes, alanine transaminase (ALT) and aspartate aminotransferase (AST) elevation, tinnitus, blurred vision, nystagmus, photosensitivity, myalgia, and dyspnea

**Severe Adverse Effects of VPA**

- VPA can lead to several severe adverse reactions, including hepatotoxicity, hallucinations, suicidality, psychosis, toxic epidermal necrolysis, Stevens-Johnson syndrome, anaphylaxis, hyponatremia, SIADH, pancreatitis, thrombocytopenia, pancytopenia, hyperammonemia, myelosuppression, hypothermia, aplastic anemia, bleeding, erythema multiforme, polycystic ovarian syndrome, cerebral pseudoatrophy, encephalopathy, and coma
- The abrupt discontinuation of the drug can trigger withdrawal seizures

**Box Warnings**

- Patients younger than 2 are at elevated risk for hepatotoxicity
- Anticonvulsant polytherapy is associated with an elevated risk of fatality
- In older patients, hepatotoxicity may present with symptoms of weakness, lethargy, anorexia, facial edema, vomiting, and loss of seizure control
- VPA use can cause life-threatening pancreatitis
- VPA can cause severe congenital malformations, including NTDs, which result in lower IQ scores when exposed in utero

## Pearls

- *Valproic acid notably decreased the occurrence and intensity of seizures in most patients without causing significant adverse effects*
- *Screening procedures should be conducted for patients to detect signs of depression, alterations in behavior, and suicidality*
- *When hypoalbuminemia is present, assessing valproate's free levels is essential due to its protein-binding nature, as the total concentration measurements may be inaccurate*
- *Acute VPA toxicity can lead to central nervous system (CNS) depression, metabolic acidosis, hypernatremia, hypoglycemia, hyperammonemia, hepatotoxicity, pancreatitis, or multiorgan failure*
- *Hepatotoxicity can be evident through elevated liver enzymes*
- *The initial step to managing VPA toxicity is discontinuing the medication*

Mood Stabilizers

# Carbamazepine (Tegretol)

## Dosage Variations

- Conventional tablets (100mg, 200mg)
- Extended-release tablets (100mg, 200mg, 300mg, and 400mg), suspensions, and cannot be crushed or chewed.

## Mechanism of Action

**Classification (Anticonvulsants):** Carbamazepine modulates voltage-gated sodium channels (VGSC), causing inhibition of action potentials and decreased synaptic transmission. Similar to other anti-convulsions, carbamazepine is suggested to bind to the alpha subunit of VGSC, specifically at a binding pocket formed by the external pore loop and the pore-lining part of domain IV.

## Indications

- **Epilepsy**
- **It is not indicated for absence seizures**
- **Trigeminal Neuralgia**
- **Acute manic and mixed episodes in bipolar I disorder**

***Off-label*** *for refractory schizophrenia, treating restless leg syndrome, decreasing agitation and aggression in patients with dementia, neuropathic pain and fibromyalgia*

## Pharmacokinetics

- Peak serum time: 4.5 hr (immediate-release tablets); 3-12 hr (extended-release tablets); 1.5 hr (oral suspension)
- Metabolized via hepatic CYP3A4
- Half-life: 25-65 hr (initial dosing); decreases to 10-20 hr after autoinduction; 35-40 hr (extended release)
- Excretion: Urine

## Adverse Effects/Contraindications

- The most common side effects of include dizziness, drowsiness, ataxia, nausea, and vomiting
- Strong association between the HLA-B*1502 gene and Steven Johnson syndrome/toxic epidermal necrolysis (SJS/TEN) -people of Asian decent
- Black box warning on agranulocytosis and aplastic anemia
- Can increase the risk of delirium in the elderly Due to the mild anticholinergic activity. This effect can also lead to urinary retention, increased intraocular pressure, and constipation.

## Pearls

- *It can cross the placenta, and this drug can also be transferred through breast milk in nursing infants, prompting the need to decide whether to discontinue nursing or discontinue the drug in the mother*
- *Anticholinergic effect can also lead to urinary retention, increased intraocular pressure, and constipation*
- *Therapy should stop if a low white blood count or platelet count appears on subsequent lab results*
- *Liver enzymes require an assessment to avoid acute liver failure*
- *Patients with increased intraocular pressure should have periodic eye examinations to look out for specific ocular changes, focusing on the slit lamp, fundoscopy, and tonometry*
- *Clinicians should discontinue this drug at the first sign of a drug-related rash, any evidence of significant bone marrow depression, or worsening hepatic damage*
- *Seizures caused by carbamazepine poisoning should receive treatment with benzodiazepines such as diazepam*

Mood Stabilizers

# Lamotrigine (Lamictal)

## Dosage Variations

- Tablet form 25mg, 100mg, 150mg, and 200 mg
- A chewable tablet 2mg, 5mg, and 25mg
- Disintegrating tablets 25mg, 50mg, 100mg, and 200mg
- All formulations should be stored at room temperature and need protection from light

## Mechanism of Action

**Classification (Phenyltriazine Antiepileptic):** The mechanism of action for lamotrigine is not entirely understood. It is a triazine, and research has shown that Lamotrigine selectively binds and inhibits voltage-gated sodium channels, stabilizing presynaptic neuronal membranes and inhibiting presynaptic glutamate and aspartate release.

## Indications

- **Seizure/Epilepsy**

***Off-label*** *rapid-cycling bipolar depression, bipolar disorder type I maintenance, prophylaxis for basilar migraine with aura, panic disorder, and binge eating disorder*

## Pharmacokinetics

- Peak plasma time: 1-1.5 hr (immediate release); 4-11 hr (extended release)
- Excretion: Renal
- Half life: 25-33 hr (adults); 25-43 hr (elderly)
- 28-116 hr + (moderate hepatic impairment);

## Adverse Effects/Contraindications

- Rash severity varies but includes a risk for Stevens-Johnson syndrome
- Other serious adverse effects include multi-organ sensitivity, hemophagocytic lymphohistiocytosis, blood dyscrasias, suicidal behavior/ideations, aseptic meningitis, status epilepticus, and sudden unexplained death in epilepsy

**Side Effects**

- Nausea, vomiting
- Chest pain, back pain
- Xerostomia
- Edema
- Dysmenorrhea
- Weight changes
- Constipation
- Abdominal pain
- Pain, weakness
- Insomnia, drowsiness
- Dizziness, ataxia, diplopia.
- Headache
- Anxiety, irritability
- Visual disturbances

## Pearls

- *Labs should include pertinent serum levels of concurrent anticonvulsants, liver function testing, and renal function assessments*
- *Patients should also monitor for changes in suicidality, including suicidal thoughts and increased desire to commit suicide*
- *Patients should receive counsel on how to watch for signs/symptoms of aseptic meningitis.*
- *Overdose at 16 g, fatalities have occurred following complications, including seizures, coma, and conduction abnormalities.*
- *There is no known specific antidote for lamotrigine toxicity*

Mood Stabilizers

# Oxcarbazepine (Trileptal)

## Dosage Variations

Only available in the oral dosage form at this time; both tablets and liquid formulations. The usual dose range is 1200mg to 2400mg per day.

## Mechanism of Action

**Classification (Anticonvulsant):** Oxcarbazepine binds to sodium channels and inhibits high-frequency repetitive neuronal firing. Oxcarbazepine also inhibits the release of glutamate. This medication gets metabolized by the liver and excreted by the kidneys. Oxcarbazepine rapidly converts to licarbazepine, its active metabolite (monohydroxy metabolite, MHD)

## Indications

- **Partial seizures in adults with epilepsy**
- **Partial seizures in children**
  - with epilepsy ages 4 to 16

**Off-label** to treat trigeminal neuralgia in patients with multiple sclerosis and bipolar disorder

## Pharmacokinetics

- Peak serum time: 4-6 hr
- Enzymes induced: CYP3A4
- Enzymes inhibited: CYP2C19
- Half-life: 2 hr (immediate-release parent drug); 9 hr (immediate-release derivative MHD); 7-11 hr (extended-release parent drug); 9-11 hr (extended-release derivative MHD)
- Excretion: Urine

## Adverse Effects/Contraindications

- It can lead to central nervous system (CNS) side effects due to its blockade of voltage-sensitive sodium channels
- Some common side effects are sedation, dizziness, abnormal gait, headache, ataxia, fatigue, confusion, nausea, vomiting, abdominal pain, or rash
- Weight gain and sedation can occur as well in a minority of patients.
- Can possibly exacerbate myoclonus in patients, and it appeared to induce absence seizures in a patient with Rasmussen syndrome
- It can cause major congenital malformations, liver injury (rarely), and movement disorder

## Pearls

- *It is essential to monitor serum sodium concentrations*
- *Approved for use in children four years and older as monotherapy or adjunctive therapy for partial seizures*
- *It can cross the placenta*
- *Breast Milk concentrations are low, and infants older than two months are expected not to cause any adverse effects*
- *For the elderly should be started at lower doses and titrated more slowly as Oxcarbazepine undergoes renal excretion*
- *Toxicity cannot be generalized to human patients*

Mood Stabilizers

# Topiramate (Topamax)

## Dosage Variations

Available in immediate-release (taken twice daily) and extended-release (taken once daily)

## Mechanism of Action

**Classification (Anticonvulsants):** (AEDs) Class: generally used for neurologic and psychiatric purposes. Although the precise mechanism of action of topiramate is unknown, there is sufficient evidence to explain the drug's anticonvulsant activity. Topiramate blocks voltage-gated sodium channels, most likely leading to sustained depolarization control during seizures. Topiramate reduces membrane depolarization by AMPA/Kainate receptors.

## Indications

- **Generalized onset tonic-clonic or partial-onset seizures**
- **For migraine disorders - prophylaxis, topiramate has been approved for prophylaxis in adults**

**Off-label** uses for topiramate, including neuropathic pain, psychotropic drug-induced weight gain, alcohol use disorders with tobacco dependence, cluster headache prevention, binge eating disorder, bulimia nervosa, obesity with hypertension, prevention of neuralgiform attacks, adjunctive therapy in bipolar disorder, unipolar depression, borderline personality disorder, obsessive-compulsive disorder, posttraumatic stress disorder, Tourette syndrome, Prader-Willie syndrome, essential tremor

## Pharmacokinetics

- Peak plasma levels usually achieved in 2 to 3 hours
- Eliminated by renal excretion
- The half-life is approximately 21 hours

## Adverse Effects/Contraindications

- Acute myopia and secondary angle-closure glaucoma
- Oligohidrosis and hyperthermia: uncommon and reversible with cessation of the drug
- Metabolic acidosis
- Suicidal behavior and ideation
- Cognitive/neuropsychiatric adverse reactions: influence of topiramate on the hippocampus-related memory processes influence spatial memory but does not significantly affect the learning process
- Fetal toxicity: Exposure during pregnancy is associated with congenital malformations and developmental delay
- Kidney stones: long term topiramate administration could induce urolithiasis
- Hepatotoxicity
- The most common adverse effects in epilepsy trials included the involvement of the central nervous system (paresthesia, fatigue, cognitive problems, dizziness, somnolence, psychomotor slowing, memory/concentration difficulties, nervousness, confusion), endocrine/metabolism (weight loss, anorexia), respiratory (infection), miscellaneous (fever, flushing)
- The most common adverse effects in trials involving migraine patients were paresthesia and dysgeusia
- alcohol should be avoided 6 hours before and after the administration

## Pearls

- *Baseline and periodic serum bicarbonate levels are required monitoring protocols for individuals on topiramate due to concern for metabolic acidosis*
- *Renal function tests should be monitored*
- *Monitoring topiramate levels is advised in special cases requiring weight-based dose adjustments in young children, patient adherence, polypharmacy, and suspected toxicity*
- *Monitor for a reduction in the frequency of the most debilitating seizures (drop attacks and tonic-clonic seizures) when topiramate is used for Lennox-Gastaut syndrome (LGS)*
- *A sprinkle capsule formulation may add to a small amount of soft food.*
- *Symptoms of toxicity include sedation, speech disturbance, blurred vision, agitation, ataxia, convulsions, and abdominal pain. ABG analysis in topiramate overdose usually demonstrates hyperchloraemic normal anion gap metabolic acidosis*

Section 3

# Antipsychotics (FGAs & SGAs)

Antipsychotics

# Aripiprazole (Abilify)

## Dosage Variations

Oral tablets, disintegrating tablets (10mg and 15mg), oral solution, and intramuscular (IM) injections (9.75mg/1.3mL) Oral dosing ranges from 5mg to 30mg/day and is available in 2mg, 5mg, 10mg, 15mg, 20mg, and 30mg tablets

## Mechanism of Action

**Classification (Atypical Antipsychotics):** Aripiprazole is a quinolinone antipsychotic that is a partial agonist at the D2 and 5HT-1a receptors and an antagonist at the 5HT-2a receptor. It has a high affinity for D2, D3, 5HT-1a, and 5HT2a receptors and moderate affinity for D4, 5HT-2c, 5-HT7, alpha-1 adrenergic, and H1 receptors. Aripiprazole has no affinity for muscarinic receptors at recommended doses.

## Indications

- Atypical antipsychotic
- Psychosis in patients with schizophrenia
- Acute manic episodes associated with bipolar disorder
- Autistic spectrum disorder (ASD)
- Major depressive disorder
- Tourette syndrome (oral tablet or oral solution only)

**Off-label:** patients with comorbid psychotic disorders and substance use disorders, delirium and apraxia of eyelid opening with blepharospasm in Parkinson disease

## Pharmacokinetics

- Peak plasma time: 1-3 hr (IR); 5-7 hr (ER); 3-5 hr (tablet);
- Protein bound: 99%
- Metabolized by CYP2D6 and CYP3A4
- Half-life: 75 hr (parent drug)
- Excretion: Feces

## Adverse Effects/Contraindications

- EPS such as akathisia, parkinsonian features such as resting tremor and shuffling gait, acute dystonic reactions, oculogyric crises, opisthotonos, and tardive dyskinesia are manageable with benztropine or sodium benzoate
- Associated with lower incidences of weight gain, hypercholesterolemia, glucose dysregulation, cardiovascular abnormalities, and hyperprolactinemia.
- Other possible side effects include somnolence, nausea, vomiting, akathisia, and lightheadedness
- Rare adverse effects may include neuroleptic malignant syndrome, liver function abnormalities and jaundice, seizures, and agranulocytosis.
- FDA boxed warning for increased risk of cerebrovascular events and death in elderly patients with psychosis related to the major neurocognitive disorder and suicidal thoughts among children, adolescents, and young adults

## Pearls

- *Patients require close monitoring for any side effects*
- *It is essential to establish baseline measurements of blood pressure (repeat in three months and annually), weight (remeasure at weeks 4, 8, and 12), height, BMI, waist circumference, electrolytes, liver function, fasting plasma glucose concentration (repeat in three months and annually), lipid panel, abnormal involuntary movement scale (repeat weekly for two weeks after initiation or dose increase), and ocular exam findings*
- *Monitor the patient's CBC frequently during the first few months in patients with preexisting leukopenia or neutropenia*
- *Closely monitor serum sodium with initiation or dosage adjustment in older adults*
- *Monitor electrolytes, liver function, changes in menstruation, libido, or other manifestations of hyperprolactinemia*
- *There is currently no known antidote for aripiprazole overdose*
- *Children and adolescents are more susceptible than older patients to experience EPS, weight gain, and other metabolic side effects*

Antipsychotics

# Brexpiprazole (Rexulti)

## Dosage Variations

Tablet forms available in 1mg, 2mg and 4mg once daily. Max dose is 4mg

## Mechanism of Action

**Classification (Atypical Antipsychotics):** It is currently known for use in schizophrenia and MDD. A suggested mechanism related to partial agonism of 5-HT1A and D2 receptors and antagonism of 5-HT2A may mediate its efficacy. Brexpiprazole is an atypical antipsychotic and a novel D2 dopamine and serotonin 1A partial agonist called serotonin-dopamine activity modulator (SDAM). It has a high affinity for serotonin, dopamine and alpha (α)-adrenergic receptors. Although it is structurally similar to aripiprazole, brexpiprazole has different binding affinities for dopamine and serotonin receptors.

## Indications

- Schizophrenia
- Adjunctive treatment with antidepressants for MDD
- Agitation associated with dementia due to Alzheimers

## Pharmacokinetics

- Absorbed in the gastrointestinal tract, and within four hours, peak plasma concentrations can be seen
- Mainly metabolized by cytochrome P450 (CYP) 2D6 and CYP3A4 and has demonstrated no effect on inducing or inhibiting any CYP 450 isoenzymes
- Excreted mostly in feces

## Adverse Effects/Contraindications

- MDD patients experiences akathisia, weight gain, constipation, fatigue, somnolence, headache, tremor, dizziness, anxiety and restlessness
- Schizophrenia patients experience a higher incidence of akathisia, tremor, sedation, dyspepsia, and weight gain, diarrhea and increased blood creatine phosphokinase
- Increased risk of mortality in elderly patients with dementia-related psychosis
- Suicidal Ideations increase with youth and young adults
- Motor/cognitive impairment, neutropenia, leukopenia, and agranulocytosis should be monitored

## Pearls

- *Dosage adjustments are necessary in patients with hepatic or renal impairment*
- *Possible change in behavior should be understood*

Antipsychotics

# Cariprazine (Vraylar)

## Dosage Variations

Dosage Forms & Strengths
capsule
- 1.5mg
- 3mg
- 4.5mg
- 6mg

## Mechanism of Action

**Classification (Atypical Antipsychotics):** Precise mechanism by which Cariprazine works for schizophrenia or bipolar disorder is unknown

Efficacy could be mediated through a combination of partial agonist activity at central dopamine (D2) and serotonin 5-HT1A receptors

## Indications

- Schizophrenia in adults
- Indicated for acute treatment of manic or mixed episodes associated with bipolar I disorder
- Indicated for treatment of depressive episodes associated with bipolar I disorder
- Indicated as adjunctive therapy to antidepressants for treatment of major depressive disorder (MDD)

## Pharmacokinetics

- Extensively metabolized by CYP3A4 to DCAR and DDCAR
- Half-life: 2-4 days
- Excretion: urine

## Adverse Effects/Contraindications

Schizophrenia
- Extrapyramidal symptoms, all (24-33)
- Extrapyramidal symptoms, excluding akathisia/ restlessness (15-20)
- Parkinsonism (13-18)
- Headache (9-18)
- Akathisia (9-14)
- Insomnia (11-13)
- Constipation (6-10)
- Somnolence (5-10)
- Nausea (5-8)
- Abdominal pain (3-7)
- Restlessness (4-6)
- Anxiety (3-6)
- Toothache (3-6)
- Hypertension (2-7)
- Dyspepsia (4-5)
- Vomiting (4-5)
- Dizziness (3-5)
- Agitation (3-5)
- Diarrhea (1-5)
- Pain in extremity (2-4)
- Cough (1-4)
- Tachycardia (2-3)
- Increased weight (2-3)
- Decreased appetite (1-3)
- Dry mouth (1-3)
- Fatigue (1-3)
- Increased CPK (1-3)
- Musculoskeletal stiffness (<3)
- Back pain (1-3)
- Dystonia (2)
- Tachycardia (1-2)
- Arthralgia (1-2)
- Hepatic enzyme increased (1-2)
- Nasopharyngitis (1-2)
- Urinary tract infections (1-2)
- Rash (1-2)

Bipolar mania
- Vomiting (8-10)
- Insomnia (8-9)
- Dyspepsia (7-9)
- Somnolence (7-8)
- Abdominal pain (6-8)
- Restlessness (7)
- Dizziness (6-7)
- Diarrhea (5-6)
- Hypertension (4-5)
- Fatigue (4-5)
- Dystonia (3-5)
- Blurred vision (4)
- Decreased appetite (3-4)
- Toothache (3-4)
- Pain in extremity (2-4)
- Pyrexia (1-4)
- Weight increased (2-3)
- Increased CPK (2-3)
- Dry mouth (2-3)
- Oropharyngeal pain (1-3)
- Back pain (1-3)
- Hepatic enzymes increased (1-3)
- Musculoskeletal stiffness (2)
- Tachycardia (1-2)
- Extrapyramidal symptoms, all (41-45)
- Extrapyramidal symptoms, excluding akathisia/restlessness (26-29)
- Parkinsonism (21-26)
- Akathisia (20-21)
- Headache (13-14)
- Nausea (11-13)
- Constipation (6-11)

Bipolar depression
- Insomnia (7-10)
- Akathisia (6-10)
- Nausea (7)
- Somnolence (6-7)
- Restlessness (2-7)
- Extrapyramidal symptoms, excluding akathisia/restlessness (4-6)
- Dizziness (3-4)
- Fatigue (3-4)
- Parkinsonism (3-4)
- Increased appetite (3)
- Increased weight (2)
- Musculoskeletal stiffness (≤1)
- Extrapyramidal symptoms, all (10-19)

MDD (cariprazine and antidepressant therapy)
- Akathisia (7-23)
- Extrapyramidal symptoms (5-18)
- Insomnia (14-16)
- Nausea (7-13)
- Somnolence (5-11)
- Fatigue (3-10)
- Insomnia (9-10)
- Restlessness (4-8)
- Nausea (6-7)
- Dizziness (4-5)
- Dry mouth (3-5)
- Constipation (2-5)
- Increased appetite (2-5)
- Blurred vision (1-4)
- Nasopharyngitis (1-4)
- Agitation (<3)
- Weight increased (2-3)
- Back pain (2-3)
- Vomiting (1-3)
- Anxiety (1-3)
- Blurred vision (<2)
- Palpitations (<2)
- Hyperhidrosis (1-2)
- Edema (1-2)
- Myalgia (1-2)

## Pearls

- *Avoid St. John's Wort. This herb induces the CYP3A metabolism of brexpiprazole and may reduce its serum concentration. The dose of Brexpiprazole should be doubled if administered with St. John's wort.*
- *Drink plenty of fluids.*
- *Take with or without food.*

Antipsychotics

# Chlorpromazine (Thorazine)

## Dosage Variations

- Tablets (10mg, 25mg, 50mg, 100mg, and 200mg). Max dose per oral is 800mg/day
- Intramuscular or intravenous route 25mg, followed as needed by 25mg to 50mg after 1 to 4 hours. The usual dose can be 300mg-800mg/day

## Mechanism of Action

**Classification (Conventional Antipsychotics):** Chlorpromazine is a member of the typical antipsychotic or neuroleptic drug class, also known as first-generation antipsychotics (FGAs). Its precise mechanism of action is unknown, but it is believed to produce its antipsychotic effect by the post-synaptic blockade at the D2 receptors in the mesolimbic pathway. However, blocking D2 receptors in the nigrostriatal pathway is responsible for its extrapyramidal side effects.

## Indications

- Schizophrenia (primarily the positive symptoms)
- Bipolar I acute manic type of manic-depressive illness
- Acute agitation marked by explosive hyperexcitable behavior out of proportion to the initial provocation
- Persistent singultus (chronic hiccups)
- Relief of apprehension before surgery
- Adjunct treatment of tetanus
- Acute intermittent porphyria

**Off-label:** Adjunct treatment of serotonin syndrome, migraine-associated relief of nausea and vomiting

## Pharmacokinetics

- Extensively metabolized by the liver (CYP450 enzymes 1A2 and 2D6; it is a CYP3A4 substrate)
- It also undergoes metabolism in the kidney and GI tract
- It is excreted in the urine, bile, and feces
- It has a half-life of between 23 and 37 hours for the parent drug

## Adverse Effects/Contraindications

- Low-potency antipsychotic that mainly causes non-neurologic side effects
- It is highly lipid-soluble and stored in body fats, thus very slow to be removed from the body
- Primarily causes dry mouth, dizziness, urine retention, blurred vision, and constipation by blocking the muscarinic receptors
- There is a risk of angle-closure glaucoma in older patients
- Decreased libido in both genders
- In males, increased prolactin may cause gynecomastia, galactorrhea, and erectile dysfunction
- Rarely, it may cause priapism
- In females, increased prolactin levels may result in irregular menstruation, oligomenorrhea, amenorrhea, and galactorrhea
- When administered as intramuscular or intravenous injections, it may cause hypotension and headache
- The drug-induced hepatotoxicity results from inflammation and injury to the liver, which may significantly increase the alanine aminotransferase level (ALT)

## Pearls

- *Patients receiving chronic treatment with chlorpromazine have lower plasma levels as compared to the patients acutely treated with an oral dose of chlorpromazine*
- *It also causes sedation due to the blockade of histamine H1 receptors*
- *Chlorpromazine use also requires caution in patients with cerebrovascular and cardiovascular diseases*
- *Treatment should be discontinued if the patient develops agranulocytosis*
- *In the event of an overdose, ensure adequate ventilation*
- *No specific antidote is available, and treatment primarily addresses symptoms with regular cardiac and respiratory monitoring*
- *In case of the early detection of liver injury, the drug should be stopped*

## Dosage Variations

- Oral tablet dosages of 25mg, 50mg, 100mg, and 200mg
- Orally disintegrating tablet dosages of 12.5mg, 25mg, 100mg, 150mg, and 200mg
- Oral suspension dosage of 50mg/mL (100mL)

Antipsychotics

# Clozapine (Clozaril)

## Mechanism of Action

**Classification (Atypical Antipsychotics):** Clozapine is part of a group of drugs known as second-generation antipsychotics or atypical antipsychotics. Antipsychotic drugs are vital in treating the core symptoms of schizophrenia: hallucinations and delusions. As an atypical antipsychotic, clozapine is an antagonist to dopamine and serotonin receptors. Clozapine binds to the dopamine D4 receptor with a higher affinity than the dopamine D2 receptor, contributing to decreased adverse events and extrapyramidal symptoms.

## Indications

- Schizophrenia
  - not first line due to adverse effects
- Schizophrenia-associated suicide prevention

## Pharmacokinetics

- Peak plasma concentrations: 2.5 hours
- First pass is liver
- Clozapine is extensively metabolized in the liver by cytochrome P450 isozymes, particularly CYP1A2, CYP2D6, and CYP3A4.
- Half-life: 8 to 12 hours
- Excretion is urine

## Adverse Effects/Contraindications

- The risk of developing agranulocytosis which may cause death
- The common adverse events associated with clozapine overdose are hypersalivation, tachycardia, hypotension, sedation, delirium, coma, respiratory depression, or failure
- Clozapine-induced myocarditis is a rare complication
- Clozapine is associated with significant weight gain, type 2 diabetes, diabetic ketoacidosis, and increased lipid levels due to increased insulin resistance
- It may lower the seizure threshold in patients with epilepsy
- Sialorrhea is a dose-dependent and benign condition that may bother some patients. One risk of excessive salivation is aspiration pneumonia
- Cholinergic and serotonergic properties of clozapine may affect the gastrointestinal system and lead to constipation or even ileus
- Laboratory abnormalities may include reduced serum iron levels, metabolic acidosis, and coagulopathy

## Pearls

- *Weekly complete blood count (CBC) to measure ANC levels*
- *Diet and exercise, blood glucose levels needed fot metabolic syndrome*
- *Baseline troponin I or T levels, high sensitivity CRP levels, echocardiography, and BNP levels, as well as vitals and weekly laboratory testing of troponins, CRP, and BNP levels*
- *Monitor EEG and clozapine blood levels for patient who seizures*
- *Lower risk for tardive dyskinesia*
- *Improvement of cognition, which leads to improved quality of life*
- *Decreased relapse*

## Dosage Variations

- Oral tablets ( 1mg, 2.5mg, 5mg, or 10mg )
- Intramuscular injections for acute symptoms, and long-acting intramuscular or subcutaneous injections
- Liquid oral solutions available for patients that are unable to tolerate tablet formulations.

Antipsychotics

# Fluphenazine (Prolixin)

## Mechanism of Action

**Classification (Antipsychotics):** Fluphenazine acts primarily through antagonism of postsynaptic dopamine-2 receptors in mesolimbic, nigrostriatal, and tuberoinfundibular neural pathways. The blockage of postsynaptic dopamine-2 receptors in the mesolimbic pathway targets positive symptoms in schizophrenia, such as hallucinations, delusions, and disorganized speech. It is also known to have antagonistic properties at alpha-1 adrenergic receptors, contributing to its cardiac and orthostatic side effects.

## Indications

- Psychosis in patients with schizophrenia
- Maintenance therapy for chronic schizophrenia and related psychotic disorders in patients
  - who do not tolerate oral formulations or in patients where medication compliance is of concern

**Off-label** use to augmentation of mood stabilization or treating concomitant psychotic symptoms in patients with bipolar disorder as well as to manage chronic tic disorders and Huntington disease to control abnormal movements and chorea, depression, tourette syndrome

## Pharmacokinetics

- Peak plasma time: 2 hr
- Half-life: 14-16hr
- Excretion: Urine, feces

## Adverse Effects/Contraindications

- Common side effects include sedation, dry mouth, dry eyes, blurred vision, constipation, orthostasis, dizziness, hypotension, and urinary retention, rebound tachycardia, urinary retention, and weight gain.
- Due to dopaminergic antagonism, fluphenazine can cause extrapyramidal symptoms, including akathisia, parkinsonian features such as resting tremor and shuffling gait, acute dystonic reactions, oculogyric crises, opisthotonos, and tardive dyskinesia can occur
- Rare but serious side effects include neuroleptic malignant syndrome, liver function abnormalities and jaundice, seizures, and agranulocytosis
- Black-box warning for increased risk of cerebrovascular events and death in elderly patients with psychosis related to the major neurocognitive disorder

## Pearls

- *Require close monitoring for the appearance of side effects*
- *Baseline electrocardiograms should be obtained in all patients with preexisting cardiac conduction abnormalities*
- *Clinicians should routinely obtain complete blood counts and metabolic panels to monitor for changes in white blood cell counts, liver transaminases, and blood urea nitrogen and creatinine levels*
- *Avoid alcohol*
- *Take with food. Food reduces irritation*
- *There is no specific antidote for toxicity; treatment is symptomatic, usually based on the presenting anticholinergic effects*
- *Opisthotonus is defined as a dramatic abnormal posture due to spastic contraction of the extensor muscles of the neck, trunk, and lower extremities*

Antipsychotics

# Haloperidol (Haldol)

## Dosage Variations

- Tablet (0.5mg, 1mg, 2mg, 5mg, 10mg, 20mg)
- Oral concentrate (2mg/mL)
- Injectable solution, lactate (5mg/mL)
- Injectable solution, decanoate (50mg/mL, 100mg/mL)

## Mechanism of Action

**Classification (Conventional Antipsychotics):** Haloperidol, a first-generation typical antipsychotic, exerts its antipsychotic effects by blocking dopamine D2 receptors in the brain. This drug reaches its maximum effectiveness when 72% of dopamine receptors are blocked. Haloperidol's effects are not limited to the D2 receptor, as it also exerts blocking action on noradrenergic, cholinergic, and histaminergic receptors. The blocking of these receptors is associated with various adverse drug reactions.

## Indications

- Schizophrenia
  - especially positive symptoms
- Tourette syndrome
- Severe behavioral disorders in children
- Hyperactivity in children

**Off-Label Uses**

- Agitation-associated with psychiatric disorders
- Chemotherapy-induced nausea and vomiting
- Management of intractable hiccups

## Pharmacokinetics

- The time to reach peak plasma concentration is around 2 to 6 hours after oral administration, 20 minutes after intramuscular (IM) administration
- First pass - Liver with involvement from CYP3A4, CYP2D6, and minor CYP1A2 enzymes
- Primarily excreted in the urine

## Adverse Effects/Contraindications

- Extrapyramidal Adverse Effects
- Acute dystonia
- Akathisia
- Neuroleptic malignant syndrome (NMS)
- Parkinsonism
- Tardive dyskinesia (TD)

**Common Adverse Effects**

- Anticholinergic effects include increased body temperature, dry mouth, drowsiness or sedation, constipation, and urinary retention
- Other common adverse effects of haloperidol include sedation, weight gain, erectile dysfunction in males, and oligomenorrhea or amenorrhea in females

**Less Common Adverse Effects**

- Orthostatic hypotension
- Lens opacities

**Rare Adverse Effects**

- cholestatic jaundice, priapism, inflammation and nodule formations with haloperidol decanoate use, and seizures

**Box Warning**

- Older patients with dementia-related psychosis have an elevated mortality risk

## Pearls

- *Monitoring of patients is crucial due to the possibility of adverse drug reactions, particularly when haloperidol is administered in the IM form*
- *Consensus guidelines for therapeutic drug monitoring (TDM) recommend a serum therapeutic range of 1 to 10 ng/mL for haloperidol*
- *As no specific antidote exists, supportive treatment is the mainstay of haloperidol toxicity*
- *If a patient shows signs of toxicity, the clinician should promptly consider performing gastric lavage or emesis induction on the patient, followed by administering activated charcoal*
- *FDA disapproves haloperidol for treating patients with dementia-related psychosis*
- *ECG and vital signs require regular monitoring, especially for signs of torsades de pointes, QT prolongation, or dysrhythmias*
- *Cardiac monitoring should be continued until the ECG returns to normal*

Antipsychotics

# Loxapine (Loxitane)

## Dosage Variations

Capsule
- 5mg
- 10mg
- 25mg
- 50mg

## Mechanism of Action

**Classification (Antipsychotics):** Dibenzoxazepine antipsychotic; blocks mesolimbic D1 and D2 receptors in the brain; also has anti-serotonin 5HT2 activity

## Indications

- Schizophrenia

This drug is not approved for the treatment of patients with dementia-related psychosis

## Pharmacokinetics

- Duration of Absorption: 12 hr
- Peak plasma time: 1-2 hr
- Half-life: 4-12 hr
- Excretion: Urine

## Adverse Effects/Contraindications

**Black Box Warnings**
- Patients with dementia-related psychosis are at an increased risk of death as shown in short-term controlled trials
- The deaths appeared to be either cardiovascular (eg, heart failure, sudden death) or infectious (eg, pneumonia) in nature

**Common**
- Hypotension, orthostatic hypotension
- Akathisia, dizziness, drug-induced tardive dystonia, dystonia, extrapyramidal disease, parkinsonian, somnolence, tardive dyskinesia
- Diminished sweating
- Constipation, xerostomia
- Blurred vision
- Urinary retention
- Nasal congestion

**Serious**
- Prolonged QT interval, torsades de pointes
- Ineffective thermoregulation, heatstroke or hypothermia (rare), neuroleptic malignant syndrome (rare), seizure (rare)
- Paralytic ileus (rare)
- Agranulocytosis (rare), disorder of hematopoietic structure (rare), leukopenia (rare), thrombocytopenia (rare)
- Cholestatic jaundice syndrome (rare)
- Drug-induced lupus erythematosus, systemic (rare)
- Priapism (rare)

## Pearls

- *The risk of falls is evident*
- *Can cause bronchospasm with potential to lead to respiratory distress and respiratory arrest*
- *Screen patients a current diagnosis, history of COPD, asthma, or other lung diseases; examine patients, including chest auscultation for respiratory signs; monitor for signs and symptoms of bronchospasm*

Antipsychotics

# Lumateperone (Caplyta)

## Dosage Variations

Administered orally, at the. FDA-approved dosage of 42mg in capsule form.

Dosages at 120 mg/day have been shown not to produce any statistically significant improvement in efficacy

## Mechanism of Action

**Classification (Atypical Antipsychotics):** Involves simultaneous modulation of dopaminergic, serotonergic, and glutamatergic neurotransmission. Its dopaminergic actions involve pre-synaptic partial agonist and post-synaptic antagonist activity at dopamine D2 receptors. This dual action at the dopamine D2 receptor is unique to lumateperone compared to other antipsychotics.

## Indications

- **Schizophrenia**
  - positive and negative symptoms
- **Bipolar depression associated with bipolar I and II disorder**
  - monotherapy or an adjunctive treatment with lithium or valproate

## Pharmacokinetics

- Peak plasma time: 1-2 hr
- Cytochrome P450 (CYP) 3A4, 2C8, and 1A2, are involved
- Half-life: ~18 hr
- Clearance: 27.9 L/hr
- Excretion: urine

## Adverse Effects/Contraindications

- Increased incidence of adverse metabolic effects, such as weight gain and hyperprolactinemia
- Likely to interact with alcohol and other sedatives as it produces sedation, especially at lower dosages
- The most common side effects are somnolence, sedation, fatigue, and constipation
- Caution those with hepatic impairment
- Will cause birth defects, miscarriage or adverse maternal or fetal outcomes
- Avoid grapefruit products
- Avoid St. John's Wort

## Pearls

- *Not approved for treatment of patients with dementia-related psychosis*
- *Interacts with glutamatergic pathways in addition to dopaminergic and serotonergic pathways*
- *Antidepressants increased the risk of suicidal thoughts and behaviors in pediatric and young adults in short-term studies*
- *Very low incidence of extrapyramidal symptoms, and potentially improved coverage of negative symptoms of schizophrenia*
- *Safety and effectiveness not established in pediatric patients*
- *Preferably taken at bedtime*
- *Avoid lumateperone in patients taking a CYP3A4 inducer or moderate to potent CYP3A4 inhibitors*
- *Those who switched to lumateperone from their current antipsychotics experienced statistically significant improvements in parameters measuring LDL-cholesterol, triglycerides, and prolactin levels*

Antipsychotics

# Lurasidone (Latuda)

## Dosage Variations

Immediate-release tablets in 20, 40, 60, 80, and 120 mg strengths

## Mechanism of Action

**Classification (Atypical Antipsychotics):** Lurasidone belongs to the benzisothiazole class. It is not fully understood but it is believed to affect both dopamine and serotonin receptors. Lurasidone is a full antagonist of dopamine D2 and serotonin 5-HT2A and 5-HT7 receptors

## Indications

- **Schizophrenia**
- **Major depressive episodes associated with bipolar depression**
    - pediatric patients (10 to 17 years of age) to treat

**off-label** to treat bipolar mania and irritability, and anger in autism spectrum disorder

## Pharmacokinetics

- Peak plasma time: 1-3 hr
- Metabolized by CYP3A4
- Half-life: 18 hr
- Excretion: Feces

## Adverse Effects/Contraindications

- Lurasidone offers a safety advantage when compared with some other atypical antipsychotic agents
- Treatment with Lurasidone has a decreased risk of metabolic side effects such as hypercholesterolemia, hyperlipidemia, hyperglycemia, and weight gain compared to Risperidone, quetiapine, and Olanzapine
- In patients with schizophrenia - nausea, akathisia, somnolence, sedation, and Parkinsonism
- In patients with bipolar depression - nausea, akathisia, headache, extrapyramidal, and sedation
- Lurasidone, when used in pregnant patients, may cause extrapyramidal or withdrawal symptoms in neonates when exposed in the third trimester

## Pearls

- *Dose monitoring is necessary for patients with renal and hepatic impairments*
- *Dose adjustment is not recommended for mild impairment but rather for moderate and severe impairment*
- *Smoking does not affect lurasidone's pharmacokinetics*
- *Lurasidone does not increase suicidal ideation or behavior*
- *FDA has issued a black box warning about the risk of death in elderly patients with dementia, there is no clinical trial data to prove this evidence*
- *There is some evidence showing high doses of lurasidone can cause small increases in TSH levels*
- *It is poorly soluble in water and after oral ingestion.*
- *There are no specific antidotes for lurasidone*

Antipsychotics

# Olanzapine (Zyprexa)

## Dosage Variations

- The tablet form is available in 2.5 mg, 5 mg, 7.5 mg, 10 mg, 15 mg, and 20 mg dosages.
- Also available in a disintegrating tablet form for those who cannot swallow.

## Mechanism of Action

**Classification (Atypical Antipsychotics):** Olanzapine is an atypical (second-generation) antipsychotic that exerts its action primarily on dopamine and serotonin receptors. It works on dopamine D2 receptors in the mesolimbic pathway as an antagonist, blocking dopamine from potential action at the post-synaptic receptor. Olanzapine binds loosely to the receptor and dissociates easily, allowing for normal dopamine neurotransmission.

## Indications

- Schizophrenia
    - if the patient is over the age of 13 years
- Bipolar I disorder, for acute treatment of manic or mixed episodes .
- Episodes of depression associated with bipolar disorder type 1 and treatment-resistant depression
- In combination with samidorphan to attenuate olanzapine-induced weight gain for schizophrenia and bipolar I disorder

Off-label Clinical Uses

- Acute agitation
- Delirium
- Anorexia nervosa
- Chemotherapy-induced nausea and vomiting (CINV)

## Pharmacokinetics

- Peak concentration is 6 hours for oral formulation and 15-45 minutes for IM formulation
- Has a half-life of 21 to 54 hours, with an average of 30 hours
- Metabolized by the liver and the cytochrome P450 system
- Excreted primarily via the renal route

## Adverse Effects/Contraindications

- Causes an increase in appetite leading to hyperphagia with a consequence of weight gain
- It should be used cautiously in patients who are obese, have little control over their food intake, and do not exercise regularly to combat weight gain
- It has a high potential to cause reduced insulin sensitivity, leading to impaired glucose tolerance, especially in a younger population
- Patients have an increased risk of developing akathisia, extrapyramidal symptoms, tardive dyskinesia, and neuroleptic malignant syndrome
- Hematological abnormalities such as neutropenia and thrombocytopenia are reported
- Reported cases of hypothermia and edema due to olanzapine
- Elderly patients with dementia who present with symptoms of psychosis should not be prescribed olanzapine due to an increased mortality risk due to increased risk of heart failure, sudden death due to cardiac causes, and pneumonia

## Pearls

- *Monitoring blood glucose levels frequently and educating patients on exercise and diet should follow a prescription for Olanzapine*
- *A serum concentration of 80mg/mL is the threshold for adverse reactions to Olanzapine*
- *Clinicians should monitor patients while discontinuing Olanzapine therapy, as there is a risk of physical withdrawal and rebound symptoms*
- *There is a risk of post-injection delirium syndrome with Olanzapine*
- *Serum concentration of Olanzapine >0.1mg/L is toxic and serum concentration>1mg/L can be fatal*
- *There is no specific antidote to olanzapine*

Antipsychotics

# Paliperidone (Invega)

## Dosage Variations

Tablet, extended release
- 1.5mg
- 3mg
- 6mg
- 9mg

IM injectable suspension prefilled syringe (once monthly, Invega Sustenna)
- 39mg
- 78mg
- 117mg
- 156mg
- 234mg

IM injectable suspension prefilled syringe (q3month, Invega Trinza)
- 273mg
- 410mg
- 546mg
- 819mg

IM injectable suspension prefilled syringe (q6month, Invega Hafyera)
- 1,092mg/3.5mL
- 1,560mg/5mL

## Mechanism of Action

**Classification (Atypical Antipsychotics):** Paliperidone palmitate is hydrolyzed to paliperidone, a major active metabolite of risperidone. Mechanism of action of paliperidone is unclear. However, its efficacy in the treatment of schizophrenia could be mediated through a combination of central dopamine D2 and serotonin 5HT2A receptor antagonism. It is believed to work by blocking the action of dopamine and serotonin receptors in the brain. This helps to regulate the activity of these neurotransmitters, which are believed to be involved in the symptoms of schizophrenia.

## Indications

- **Schizophrenia**

## Pharmacokinetics

- Peak plasma time: 24 hr
- Metabolized by CYP2D6 and CYP3A4
- Excretion: Urine

## Adverse Effects/Contraindications

- Blood and lymphatic system disorders: Anemia
- Cardiac disorders: Bradycardia, tachycardia
- Ear and labyrinth disorders: Vertigo
- Gastrointestinal disorders: Constipation, nausea, vomiting
- General disorders and administration site conditions: Fatigue
- Hepatobiliary disorders: Transaminases increased
- Metabolism and nutritional disorders: Decreased appetite, increased appetite, weight decreased
- Psychiatric disorders: Depression
- Reproductive system and breast disorders: Breast pain, menstrual disorder
- Skin and SC tissue disorders: Rash
- Vascular disorders: Hypertension

**Tablets**
- Cardiac disorders: Bradycardia, palpitations
- Eye disorders: Eye movement disorder
- Gastrointestinal disorders: Flatulence
- General disorders: Edema
- Immune system disorders: Anaphylactic reaction
- Infections and infestations: Urinary tract infection
- Investigations: ALT/AST increased
- Musculoskeletal and connective tissue disorders: Arthralgia, pain in extremity
- Nervous system disorders: Opisthotonos
- Psychiatric disorders: Agitation, insomnia, nightmare
- Reproductive system and breast disorders: Breast discomfort, menstruation irregular, retrograde ejaculation
- Respiratory, thoracic, and mediastinal disorders: Nasal congestion
- Skin and SC tissue disorders: pruritus, rash Vascular disorders: Hypertension
- Cardiac disorders: AV block first degree, bundle branch block, palpitations, postural orthostatic tachycardia syndrome
- Eye disorders: Eye movement disorder, eye rolling, oculogyric crisis, vision blurred
- Gastrointestinal disorders: Abdominal discomfort/abdominal pain upper, diarrhea, dry mouth, toothache
- General disorders and administration site conditions: Asthenia, chest discomfort
- Immune system disorders: Hypersensitivity
- Investigations: Electrocardiogram (ECG) abnormal
- Metabolism and nutrition disorders: Hyperinsulinemia
- Musculoskeletal and connective tissue disorders: Myalgia, pain in extremity, joint stiffness, muscle spasms, muscle twitching, nuchal rigidity
- Nervous system disorders: Bradykinesia, cerebrovascular accident, convulsion, dizziness, dizziness postural, dysarthria, hypertonia, lethargy, oromandibular dystonia, psychomotor hyperactivity, syncope
- Psychiatric disorders: Agitation, nightmare
- Reproductive system and breast disorders: Breast discharge, erectile dysfunction, gynecomastia, sexual dysfunction
- Respiratory, thoracic, and mediastinal disorders: Cough
- Skin and SC tissue disorders: Drug eruption, eczema, pruritus, pruritus generalized, urticaria
- Vascular disorders: Hypotension, orthostatic hypotension

**Postmarketing Reports**
- Angioedema, catatonia, ileus, somnambulism, swollen tongue, thrombotic thrombocytopenic purpura, urinary incontinence, and urinary retention
- Invega Sustenna
- Anaphylactic reactions

## Pearls

- *Not approved for use in patients with dementia-related psychosis*
- *Can cause metabolic changes such as weight gain, increased blood sugar levels, and elevated cholesterol levels.*
- *Invega should be used with caution during pregnancy, as there may be a risk to the fetus*
- *It is not recommended for use while breastfeeding, as it can pass into breast milk*
- *Stopping Invega abruptly can lead to withdrawal symptoms*

Antipsychotics

# Perphenazine (Trilafon)

## Dosage Variations

Dosage Forms & Strengths
tablets
- 2mg
- 4mg
- 8mg
- 16mg

## Mechanism of Action

**Classification (Piperazinyl Phenothiazine):** Antipsychotic that blocks postsynaptic mesolimbic dopaminergic receptors in the brain; it has moderate anticholinergic effects, weak to moderate sedative effects, strong extrapyramidal effects, and strong antiemetic activity.

## Indications

- **Treatment of Nausea/Vomiting**
- **Schizophrenia**

**Intractable Hiccoughs (Off-label)**

## Pharmacokinetics

- **Peak Plasma Time:** 1-3 hr
- **Half-Life:** 9-12 hr (; 10-19 hr (metabolite)
- **Metabolism:** Hepatic P450 enzyme CYP2D6
- **Enzymes inhibited:** CYP2D6
- **Excretion:** Urine and feces

## Adverse Effects/Contraindications

**EPS**
- Akathisia (60%)
- Dystonia
- Muscle stiffness
- Neuroleptic malignant syndrome (infrequent but serious)
- Parkinsonism
- Tardive dyskinesia

**Less Common**
- Orthostatic hypotension (post-IM inj), tachycardia
- Anxiety, agitation, cerebral edema, depression, dizziness, euphoria, headache, insomnia, restless, weakness
- Anorexia, dyspepsia, constipation, ileus
- Lens opacities (prolonged use)

**Black Box Warnings**
- Patients with dementia-related psychosis who are treated with antipsychotic drugs are at an increased risk of death
- The deaths appeared to be either cardiovascular

**Common**
- Anticholinergic effects
- Sedation
- Weight gain
- Oligomenorrhea/ amenorrhea
- Erectile dysfunction

**Uncommon**
- ECG changes
- Photosensitivity
- Pruritis
- Galactorrhea
- Ejaculatory disorder
- Diarrhea
- Blood dyscrasia

**Rare**
- Seizure
- Priapism
- Cholestatic jaundice

## Pearls

- *Avoid lactation if taking this medicine*

## Dosage Variations

Tablets

- 1mg
- 2mg

Antipsychotics

# Pimozide (Orap)

## Mechanism of Action

**Classification (Diphenylbutylpiperidine):** Phenylbutylpiperadine; potent centrally acting dopamine D2 receptor antagonist

## Indications

- **Tourette Disorder**

## Pharmacokinetics

- **Peak plasma time:** 6-8 hrs.
- **Metabolism:** Hepatic P450 enzyme CYP3A4 and CYP2D6
- **Half-life elimination:** 55 hrs.
- **Excretion:** Urine

## Adverse Effects/Contraindications

**>10%**

- Akinesia (40%)
- Drowsiness (35%)
- EPS (10-15%)
- Sedation (70%)
- Speech disorder (10-15%)
- Visual disturbance (20%)
- Dry mouth (25%)
- Constipation (20%)
- Impotence (10-15%)

**1-10%**

- Appetite increase
- Thirst increase
- Dizziness
- Drug-induced tardive dystonia
- Nervousness
- Photosensitivity
- Taste change
- Orthostatic hypotension
- Diminished sweating
- Nasal congestion
- Diarrhea
- Urinary retention
- Retinitis pigmentosa

**Frequency Not Defined**

- Ineffective thermoregulation
- Heatstroke or hypothermia (rare)
- Neuroleptic malignant syndrome (rare)
- Seizure (rare)
- Prolonged QT interval
- Torsades de pointes
- Obstipation (rare)
- Paralytic ileus (rare)
- Agranulocytosis (rare)
- Disorder of hematopoietic structure (rare)
- Leukopenia (rare)
- Thrombocytopenia (rare)
- Cholestatic jaundice syndrome (rare)
- Drug-induced lupus erythematosus, systemic (rare)
- Priapism (rare)
- Death

## Pearls

- *Neonates exposed to antipsychotic drugs during the 3rd trimester of pregnancy are at risk for extrapyramidal and/or withdrawal symptoms following delivery*
- *Avoid grapefruit juice during in medication with this drug*
- *Leukopenia/neutropenia and agranulocytosis reported*

Antipsychotics

# Quetiapine (Seroquel)

## Dosage Variations

- Tablet, immediate release ( 25mg, 50mg, 100mg, 200mg, 300mg, 400mg)
- Tablet, extended release ( 50mg, 150mg, 200mg, 300mg, 400mg)

## Mechanism of Action

**Classification (Atypical Antipsychotics):** Quetiapine has a strong affinity for the 5-HT2 receptor. Although quetiapine has many complex mechanisms, it mediates its pharmacological effect mainly via its 5HT2 antagonistic action. It also acts on dopaminergic D1 and D2 receptors. Quetiapine is an antagonist for D2 receptors and 5-HT2 receptors.

## Indications

- **Schizophrenia**
- **Acute manic episodes**
- **Major depressive disorder**
- **Treatment for acute manic episodes associated with bipolar I disorder**

**Off-label:** generalized anxiety disorder, psychosis in patients with Parkinson's disease, insomnia, maintenance of schizophrenia, and chronic post-traumatic stress disorder (PTSD), adjunctive treatment with SSRI for obsessive-compulsive disorder (OCD), borderline personality disorder, decreasing aggression with psychiatric illness, major depressive disorder, and symptomatic treatment of insomnia, agitation, and anxiety

## Pharmacokinetics

- Metabolized in liver by CYP3A4
- Half-life: Immediate release, 6 hr; extended release, 7 hr
- Excretion: Urine

## Adverse Effects/Contraindications

- Associated with an increased risk of death in dementia-related psychosis in elderly patients
- Not approved for children <10 years
- Alongside this risk, neuroleptic malignant syndrome should be a consideration due to its D2 receptor blockage
- There is an increased risk for suicidal thoughts and behavior associated with drug treatment in major depressive disorder patients
- Somnolence, orthostatic hypotension, and dizziness are the most common side effects of quetiapine
- Stroke, myocarditis, and coronary heart disease have also correlated with the use of this drug

## Pearls

- *Monitor the metabolic panel with a specific focus on fasting glucose, cholesterol and triglyceride levels, blood pressure, and weight*
- *Patients should also receive a lens examination every six months during long-term treatment for cataract monitoring*
- *Agranulocytosis is a very rare but reported side effect associated with quetiapine use*
- *Quetiapine can be life-threatening if abused or misused*
- *No definitive antidote exists to reverse quetiapine toxicity*
- *It is the least likely of atypical antipsychotics to cause extrapyramidal symptoms*

Antipsychotics

# Risperidone (Risperdal)

## Dosage Variations

- Tablet (0.25mg, 0.5mg, 1mg, 2mg, 3mg, 4mg)
- Oral solution (1mg/mL)

## Mechanism of Action

**Classification (Atypical Antipsychotics):** Has high affinity for serotonin type 2 (5-HT2) receptors; binds to dopamine D2 receptors with 20 times lower affinity than that for 5-HT2 receptors; antagonizes alpha1-adrenergic, alpha2-adrenergic, and histaminergic receptors; has moderate affinity for serotonin type 1 (5-HT1C, 5-HT1D, 5-HT1A) receptors; has weak affinity for dopamine D1 receptors; has no affinity for muscarinic, beta1-adrenergic, and beta2-adrenergic receptors.

## Indications

- Schizophrenia
  - in adults and children aged 13 and up
- Bipolar I acute manic or mixed episodes as monotherapy
  - in adults and children aged ten and up
- Bipolar I acute manic or mixed episodes adjunctive with lithium or valproate
- Autism-associated irritability
  - in children aged five and up

off-label: borderline personality, delusional disorder, delirium, depression, brain injury, pedophilia, PTSD, bipolar disorder, conduct disorder, Lesch-Nyhan, Tourette, trichotillomania, stuttering, movement disorders, and developmental disorders

## Pharmacokinetics

- Risperidone once absorbed is rapidly distribute
- Extensively metabolized by liver
- Excreted in Urine
- Half-life IM: 3-6 days

## Adverse Effects/Contraindications

- Weight changes, metabolic changes, and sedation are significant concerns with risperidone
- Increased incidence of cerebrovascular disease reported; may alter cardiac conduction; life threatenin
- May cause anticholinergic effects including blurred vision, urinary retention, agitation, confusion, blurred vision, and xerostomia
- Use with caution in patients with history of seizures, Parkinson disease, Lewy body dementia, cardiovascular disease, hypovolemia, dehydration
- Leukopenia/neutropenia and agranulocytosis reported; possible risk factors for leukopenia/neutropenia include pre existing low white blood cell (WBC) count and history of drug-induced leukopenia/neutropenia
- Serious side effects of antipsychotic medications (like risperidone) can include neuroleptic malignant syndrome (NMS)

## Pearls

- *No mandatory requirements for therapeutic drug monitoring (TDM)*
- *Therapeutic monitoring can benefit assessing compliance and identifying low drug concentrations that may be low, resulting in therapeutic failure*
- *When using risperidone, the clinician may derive patient benefit by monitoring serum prolactin level, hepatic functioning, metabolic functioning, thyroid functioning, weight/BMI, height, waist circumference, blood pressure, fasting plasma glucose, insulin, fasting lipid profile, and QTc*
- *Use with caution in children <15 kg*

Antipsychotics

# Thioridazine (Mellarill)

## Dosage Variations

- The tablets come in either 10 mg, 15mg, 25mg, 50mg, 100mg, 150mg, or 200mg. Max dose 800mg per day
- Liquid form at 30mg/mL and 100mg/mL

## Mechanism of Action

**Classification (Antipsychotic):** Typical antipsychotics, including thioridazine, work to treat psychosis by blocking dopamine (DA) receptors. These medications effectively treat the positive symptoms of schizophrenia, such as hallucinations, delusions, and disorganization. Positive symptoms are believed to manifest as a result of increased levels of dopamine in the mesolimbic pathway.

## Indications

- **Schizophrenia and schizophrenia spectrum disorders**

**Off-label** uses include depression with psychotic features, pediatric behavioral disorders, and geriatric psychoneurotic manifestations

## Pharmacokinetics

- **Half-Life elimination:** 24 hr
- **Metabolism:** Hepatic P450 enzyme CYP2D6
- **Enzymes inhibited:** CYP2D6
- **Duration:** 4-5 days

## Adverse Effects/Contraindications

- Extrapyramidal side effects include symptoms of dystonia, parkinsonism, and tardive dyskinesia
- Neuroleptic Malignant Syndrome (NMS) is another serious side effect of all antipsychotics and occurs more frequently with typical antipsychotics. This adverse effect may occur suddenly
- The provider should monitor for unstable vital signs, such as tachycardia, fever, muscle rigidity, elevated white blood cell count, and creatinine phosphokinase
- Before starting this medication, it would be wise to order an ECG and monitor QTc prolongation or other ECG changes during treatment
- The development of pigmentary retinopathy is a unique adverse manifestation associated with thioridazine and not with other antipsychotics
- There is a black-box warning for dementia-related psychosis because it may increase the risk of death secondary to cerebrovascular events in the elderly
- Patients with known heart arrhythmias or hypotensive or hypertensive heart disease should also avoid this medication

## Pearls

- *Patients require monitoring for medication side effects during treatment*
- *It is important to get a baseline ECG and potassium level*
- *Another possible side effect of thioridazine is leukopenia, and thus routine complete blood counts are recommended over the course of the initial weeks*
- *Advisable to get a pregnancy test before administering the drug*
- *Thioridazine must be cautioned for use in the third trimester of pregnancy, as it may be associated with a risk of neonatal withdrawal symptoms and extrapyramidal side effects*
- *Thioridazine is a low potency typical antipsychotic, like chlorpromazine*

Antipsychotics

# Thiothixene (Navane)

## Dosage Variations

Capsule available in (1mg, 2mg, 5mg, 10mg)

## Mechanism of Action

**Classification (Antipsychotics):** Thioxanthene; dopamine D2 receptor antagonist; may also have anticholinergic and alpha-blocking effects

## Indications

- **Schizophrenia**

## Pharmacokinetics

- **Half-life elimination:** 24 hr
- **Metabolism:** Liver (CYP1A2)

## Adverse Effects/Contraindications

**Frequency Not Defined**

- Constipation
- Decr sweating
- Drowsiness
- EPS
- Incr appetite
- Orthostatic hypotension
- Photosensitivity
- Wt gain
- Xerostomia
- Agitation
- Allergic dermatitis
- Allergic reactions
- Anorexia
- Anticholinergic effects
- Anxiety
- Cerebral edema
- Depression
- Dizziness
- Erectile dysfunction
- Euphoria
- Headache
- Ileus
- Insomnia
- Irregular menses
- Lens opacities (prolonged use)
- Poikilothermia
- Rash
- Restlessness
- Sedation
- Tachycardia
- Weakness
- Agranulocytosis, blood dyscrasias (rare)
- Galactorrhea (rare)
- Heat stroke (rare)
- NMS (infrequent but serious)
- Obstructive hyperbilirubinemia (rare)
- Cholestatic jaundice
- Confusion
- Decr gag reflex
- Gynecomastia
- Hyperpyrexia
- Peripheral edema

**Black Box Warnings**

- This drug is not approved for the treatment of patients with dementia-related psychosis
- The deaths appeared to be either cardiovascular

## Pearls

- *Drug should be given to pregnant patients only when, in the judgment of the physician, the expected benefits from treatment exceed possible risks to mother and fetus*

Antipsychotics

# Trifluoperazine (Stelazine)

## Dosage Variations

Tablet

- 1mg
- 2mg
- 5mg
- 10mg

## Mechanism of Action

**Classification (Conventional Antipsychotics):** Piperazine phenothiazine agent; antagonist for the postsynaptic mesolimbic dopaminergic D2 receptors in the brain; decreases the release of hypothalamic and hypophyseal hormones.

## Indications

- **Schizophrenia**
- **Non Psychotic Anxiety**
- **Renal Impairment**

## Pharmacokinetics

- Half-Life elimination: 24 hr
- Metabolism: Liver

## Adverse Effects/Contraindications

- Adverse effects include EPS (60%; muscle stiffness, dystonia, parkinsonism, tardive dyskinesia, akathisia), NMS (infrequent but serious), Sedation, Anticholinergic effects and weight gain
- Hypersensitivity to phenothiazines or excipients
- Comatose or greatly depressed states due to central nervous system depressants, existing blood dyscrasias, bone marrow depression, and preexisting liver damage
- Thrombocytopenia and anemia reported in patients receiving therapy; agranulocytosis and pancytopenia also reported; warn patients to report sudden appearance of sore throat or other signs of infection.

## Pearls

- *This drug is not approved for the treatment of patients with dementia-related psychosis*
- *The deaths appeared to be either cardiovascular (eg, heart failure, sudden death) or infectious (eg, pneumonia) in nature.*

Antipsychotics

# Ziprasidone (Geodon)

## Dosage Variations

- It is available as oral capsules in 20 mg, 40 mg, 60, and 80 mg strength.
- Intramuscular injection ( 20mg per mL)

## Mechanism of Action

**Classification (Atypical Antipsychotics):** Ziprasidone is an atypical antipsychotic that has a binding affinity for dopaminergic (DA), serotonergic (5HT), adrenergic (a1), and histaminergic (HA) receptors. Regarding treatment for schizophrenia, antagonism of the dopamine (D2) receptor in the mesolimbic pathway has proven efficacious in diminishing positive symptoms, whereas the antagonism of the 5HT2A receptor in the mesocortical pathway has demonstrated reduction of negative symptoms of psychosis. Its efficacy and mechanism of action for treating bipolar disorder are unknown. The antagonization of both histaminergic and adrenergic (a1) receptors can induce somnolence and orthostatic hypotension.

## Indications

- **Schizophrenia**
- **Bipolar mania**
- **Acute agitation in schizophrenic patients**

**Off-label**: acute hypomania, monotherapy as maintenance treatment for adult patients with bipolar I disorder, hyperactivity treatment, and for the treatment of delirium in the ICU

## Pharmacokinetics

- Ziprasidone has a half-life of seven hours to ten hours
- This drug will reach a steady-state concentration within one to three days of dosing
- The average systemic clearance is 7.5 ml/min/kg
- A minimal amount of ziprasidone is excreted in the urine Its elimination is primarily through the liver

## Adverse Effects/Contraindications

- Patients treated with antipsychotic drugs may develop tardive dyskinesia
- If you suspect tardive dyskinesia in a patient, discontinue the drug as there is no treatment currently available to treat this movement disorder
- If you suspect patients with neuroleptic malignant syndrome, supportive care is the most important in management
- Hyperglycemia associated with coma, ketoacidosis, or death can occur in rare cases
- Patients who have diabetes mellitus should take ziprasidone with caution
- Rare but fatal Drug Reaction with Eosinophilia and Systemic Symptoms (DRESS) has been reported with Ziprasidone exposure
- Chronic hyperprolactinemia with hypogonadism may lead to decreased bone density
- Common adverse effects were drowsiness, headache, dizziness, nausea, and lightheadedness, orthostatic hypotension, akathisia, anxiety, skin rash, weight gain, constipation, dyspepsia, xerostomia, vomiting, diarrhea, visual disturbances, and pain at the injection site
- Patients taking other drugs that act on the central nervous system (CNS) should also not be administered the drug due to additive adverse reaction potential

## Pearls

- *It carries a possible risk of causing leukopenia, neutropenia, and agranulocytosis; therefore, patients with a history of low white blood cells (WBC) or drug-induced neutropenia/leukopenia should have their complete blood count monitored in the first two months of therapy*
- *If patients have a neutrophil count of less than 1000/mm^3, the clinician must discontinue the drug until the WBC count has been fully recovered*
- *Continuous ECG monitoring should start in case an arrhythmia occurs*
- *Clinicians should exercise caution in giving ziprasidone to patients with cardiovascular disease and cerebrovascular disease. Monitor blood pressure at baseline and periodically thereafter*
- *Monitor patient weight, lipid profile, blood glucose levels at baseline and three months after starting the medicine. Additionally, electrolyte levels (potassium, magnesium) could be monitored annually and as clinically indicated*
- *Patients can develop a rash based on exposure time to the drug*
- *Charcoal is also an option, along with a laxative for drug clearance*

Section 4

# Anticholinergics/ Antihistamines/ Alpha 1 Adrenergic Blockers

Anticholinergics/Antihistamines/Alpha 1 Adrenergic Blockers

# Benztropine (Cogentin)

## Dosage Variations

- Oral Route (0.5 mg, 1 mg, and 2 mg strengths)
- Intramuscular (IM) Route (1 mg per mL injection)
- Intravenous (IV) Route (1 mg per mL injection) reserved for drug-induced extrapyramidal symptoms or whenever oral and IM administration are unsuitable

## Mechanism of Action

**Classification (Anticholinergic):** Benztropine antagonizes acetylcholine and histamine receptors. In the CNS and smooth muscles, benztropine exerts its action by competing with acetylcholine at muscarinic receptors. Consequently, it reduces central cholinergic effects by blocking muscarinic receptors that appear to improve the symptoms of Parkinson disease

## Indications

**FDA approved**

- Adjunctive therapy of all forms of parkinsonism
- Idiopathic parkinsonism
- Post-encephalitic parkinsonism
- Drug-induced extrapyramidal symptoms
- The prevention of dystonic reactions
- Acute treatment of dystonic reactions

**Off-label** use in chronic sialorrhea occurring in developmentally-disabled patients and in managing intractable hiccups

## Pharmacokinetics

- Onset: PO, 1 hr; parenteral, 15 min
- Duration: 6-48 hr
- Protein bound: 95%
- Trace amounts found unchanged in feces

## Adverse Effects/Contraindications

**Mild Adverse Effects**

- Fever
- Rash
- General weakness, lethargy, and insomnia
- Nausea and vomiting
- Headache and drowsiness
- Insomnia
- Paraesthesia
- Xerostomia
- Mydriasis

**Moderate Adverse Effects**

- Myasthenia
- Heatstroke, heat intolerance, or hyperthermia
- Visual hallucinations and delirium
- Confusion and toxic psychosis
- Depression
- Psychotic symptoms (worsening of pre-existing symptoms)
- Blurred vision
- Cycloplegia
- Impairment of memory
- Dry mouth
- Parotitis
- Dysuria and urinary tract infections
- Sinus tachycardia
- Constipation
- Numbness of fingers

**Severe Adverse Effects**

- Toxic megacolon
- Paralytic ileus
- Ocular hypertension

## Pearls

- *Geriatric patients are more sensitive and have an intense response to anticholinergic medicines*
- *It is crucial to provide sufficient clinical monitoring for benztropine administration in a relatively warm environment as it can cause anhidrosis to specific groups of patients*
- *It should be careful in alcoholic patients and patients conducting manual labor in hot and humid weather*
- *The risk assessment for benztropine overdose can take place as soon as 6 hours after ingestion, and toxicity effects may vary between 12 hours to 5 days at most*
- *Decontaminating benztropine toxicity in cooperative and alert patients can be done by administering 50 g of activated charcoal during the first 2 hours of benztropine ingestion*
- *Physostigmine is the antidote for benztropine toxicity in the event delirium is not controlled through benzodiazepines*

Anticholinergics/Antihistamines/Alpha 1 Adrenergic Blockers

# Cyproheptadine (Periactin)

## Dosage Variations

- Tablet available in 4mg
- Oral solution in 2mg/5mL

## Mechanism of Action

**Classification (Antihistamines):** Serotonin and histamine antagonist; competitively inhibits H1 (histamine) receptor, mediating bronchial constriction, smooth-muscle contraction, edema, hypotension, CNS depression, and cardiac arrhythmias; prevents histamine release in blood vessels and is more effective in preventing histamine response than in reversing it; may be useful in patients with syndromes sustained by histamine-producing tumor

## Indications

- **Hypersensitivity Reaction (Allergic reactions)**
- **Off-label** Spasticity Associated With Spinal Cord, Migraine Headache Prophylaxis, Decreased Appetite Secondary to Chronic Disease, Drug-Induced Sexual Dysfunction, Serotonin Syndrome

## Pharmacokinetics

- Peak plasma time: 6-9 hr
- Excretion: Urine

## Adverse Effects/Contraindications

- Psychiatric/neurologic: CNS depression, drowsiness, sedation ranging from mild drowsiness to deep sleep (most frequent), dizziness, lassitude, disturbed coordination; less commonly, restlessness, insomnia, tremors, euphoria, nervousness, irritability, delirium, seizures, toxic psychosis, paresthesia
- Muscular: Weakness
- Cardiovascular: Palpitation, tachycardia, palpitation, ECG changes (eg, widened QRS), arrhythmias (eg, extrasystole, heart block), hypotension, hypertension, dizziness, sedation, hypotension
- GI: Epigastric distress, anorexia, nausea, vomiting, diarrhea, constipation
- Hepatic: Cholestasis, hepatitis, hepatic failure, hepatic function abnormality, jaundice (rare)
- Skin: Eczema, pruritus, inflammation, papular rash, erythema on exposed skin
- Sensory: Visual disturbances, blurred vision, diplopia, tinnitus, acute labyrinthitis
- Renal: Dysuria, urinary retention
- Respiratory: Thickening of bronchial secretions, wheezing, nasal stuffiness

## Pearls

- *It may be acceptable for pregnant women & lactating moms*
- *Stimulates the appetite by focusing on the hypothalamus*
- *Paradoxical stimulation has been noted in pediatric patients regarding sedation*
- *Avoid alcohol*

Anticholinergics/Antihistamines/Alpha 1 Adrenergic Blockers

# Diphenhydramine (Benadryl)

## Dosage Variations

It can be given by tablet, capsule, or solution by mouth; by intramuscular (IM) or intravenous (IV) injection; or topically

## Mechanism of Action

**Classification (Antihistamines):** Diphenhydramine mainly works through antagonizing the H1 (histamine 1) receptor, although it has other mechanisms of action as well. Diphenhydramine is being investigated for its anxiolytic and anti-depressant properties.

## Indications

- **Dystonias**
- **Insomnia**
- **Pruritis**
- **Urticaria**
- **Vertigo**
- **Motion sickness**

- **Off-label** use is for the treatment of oral mucositis

## Pharmacokinetics

- Onset: 15-30 min
- Duration: ≤12 hr (histamine-induced flare suppression)
- Peak serum time: 2 hr (PO)
- Metabolized by liver (first-pass)
- Half-life: 5 hr (children); 9 hr (adults); 13.5 hr (elderly)
- Excretion: Urine

## Adverse Effects/Contraindications

**Common Adverse Effects**

- Drowsiness
- Dizziness
- Impaired coordination
- Headache
- Epigastric discomfort
- Thickened bronchial secretions
- Dry mucous membranes
- CNS stimulation, paradoxical
- Constipation
- Euphoria
- Ataxia

**Serious Reactions**

- Anaphylaxis/anaphylactoid reaction
- QT prolongation
- Anemia, hemolytic
- Thrombocytopenia
- Agranulocytosis
- Leukopenia
- Pancytopenia
- Arrhythmias
- Seizures
- Toxic psychosis
- Labyrinthitis, acute
- Heatstroke

**Cautions**

- May cause CNS depression, which can impair driving or operating heavy machinery
- May potentiate the effects of sedatives, including alcohol
- Use caution in patients with asthma, hyperthyroidism, cardiovascular disease, hypertension, or increased ocular pressure.

## Pearls

- *Obtain baseline creatinine level in pediatric patients*
- *Monitor all patients for mental alertness and relief of symptoms*
- *Store at room temperature of 15 to 30 degrees C and protect from freezing and light*
- *Overdose can cause significant toxicity, ranging from agitation to cardiac arrhythmias to rhabdomyolysis and classic anticholinergic toxidrome*
- *For treatment it may attempt activated charcoal if within 1 hour of ingestion*
- *Magnesium sulfate should be administered intravenously for prolonged QT interval*
- *No to breastfeeding mothers - crosses the barrier*

Anticholinergics/Antihistamines/Alpha 1 Adrenergic Blockers

# Hydroxyzine (Vistaril-Atarax)

## Dosage Variations

- Tablet (10mg, 25mg, 50mg)
- Capsule (25mg, 50mg, 100mg)
- Syrup/oral suspension (10mg/mL)
- Injectable solution (25 mg/mL, 50mg/mL)

## Mechanism of Action

**Classification (Antihistamines):** Prazosin is an alpha-1 adrenergic receptor antagonist. Alpha-1-receptors are present on smooth muscle, as in the blood vessel walls, the prostate, urethra, iris dilator muscle, and brain. Alpha 1 antagonists cause smooth muscle relaxation, which can, in turn, cause a decrease in blood pressure by decreasing systemic vascular resistance. This medication can also cross the blood-brain barrier

## Indications

**FDA approved**

- Anxiety and Tension
- typically associated with psychoneuroses
- Pruritus
- Chronic Urticaria

**Off-label:** Nausea & Vomiting

## Pharmacokinetics

- Onset: 15-30 min (PO)
- Duration: Sedation, 4-6 hr; antipruritic, 1-12 hr; histamine-induced wheal and flare, 2-36 hr
- Peak serum time: 1-2 hr
- Distribution: Vd: 16 L/kg (adults); 23 L/kg (elderly)
- Metabolized: by liver
- Half-life: 20 hr (adults); 29 hr (elderly); 37 hr (hepatic dysfunction)
- Excretion: Urine

## Adverse Effects/Contraindications

**Common side effects**

- Sedation
- Impairment of motor function
- Confusion
- Dizziness
- Blurred vision
- Dry mouth and throat
- Palpitations
- Tachycardia
- Abdominal distress
- Constipation
- Headache

**Contraindications**

- Documented hypersensitivity or related product including cetirizine and levocetirizine and components of the formulation
- Prolonged QT interval
- SC, intra-arterial, or IV administration

## Pearls

- *This medication does not require routine drug monitoring*
- *Reported to prolong the QT/QTc interval based on postmarketing reports of rare events of Torsade de Pointes, cardiac arrest, and sudden death, and should be used with caution in patients with an increased baseline risk for QTc prolongation*
- *Hydroxyzine may potentiate the effects of central nervous system (CNS) depressants following general anesthesia*
- *Antihistamines can worsen urinary retention and glaucoma*

## Dosage Variations

Oral medication available in 1 mg capsule, 2 mg capsule, and a 5 mg capsule

Anticholinergics/Antihistamines/Alpha 1 Adrenergic Blockers

# Prazosin (Minipress)

## Mechanism of Action

**Classification (Alpha-Blockers):** Prazosin inhibits the postsynaptic alpha-1 adrenoceptors. This inhibition blocks the vasoconstricting (narrowing) effect of catecholamines (epinephrine and norepinephrine) on the vessels, leading to peripheral blood vessel dilation. Through blood vessel constriction by adrenergic receptor activation, epinephrine and norepinephrine normally act to increase blood pressure.

## Indications

**FDA Approved**

- Prazosin
- treatment of hypertension alone or in combination with other antihypertensive agents

***Non-FDA Approved/Off-label Use***

- (BPH), post-traumatic stress disorder (PTSD) associated nightmares, Raynaud phenomenon, pheochromocytoma, and scorpion envenomation.

## Pharmacokinetics

- Metabolize: CYP450 enzymes hepatically
- Half-life: is approximately 2.5 hours

## Adverse Effects/Contraindications

**Serious Adverse Effects**

- First dose hypotension
- Orthostatic hypotension
- Intraoperative Floppy iris syndrome
- Priapism
- Syncope
- Dizziness
- Headache
- Drowsiness
- Lack of energy
- Weakness
- Palpitations
- Nausea
- Vomiting
- Diarrhea
- Constipation
- Edema
- Orthostatic hypotension
- Dyspnea
- Syncope
- Vertigo
- Depression
- Rash
- Urinary frequency
- Nasal congestion
- Vertigo
- Nervousness

**Rare Side Effects**

- Abdominal pain
- Tachycardia
- Paresthesias
- Hallucinations
- Pruritus
- Incontinence
- Impotence and priapism

## Pearls

- *Increased risk of orthostatic hypotension*
- *No routine monitoring needed*
- *If you experience any serious side effects like fainting (syncope), weakness, rapid heartbeat (tachycardia), difficulty getting or keeping an erection (impotence), or severe dizziness upon standing (orthostatic hypotension), consult your healthcare provider.*
- *Prazosin itself is not typically toxic*
- *High doses or overdoses can cause significant blood pressure drop (hypotension)*

Section 5

# Stimulants

Stimulants

# Amphetamine (Dextroamphetamine)

## Dosage Variations

- Extended-release capsule: 5mg, 10mg, 15mg, 20mg, 25mg, 30mg
- Tablet: 5mg, 7.5mg, 10mg, 12.5mg, 15mg, 20mg, 30mg

## Mechanism of Action

**Classification (CNS):** Amphetamines are non-catecholamines, sympathomimetic amines with central nervous system (CNS) stimulant activity. Amphetamines increase dopamine and norepinephrine in the synaptic space by promoting the release of catecholamines from the presynaptic nerve terminals. They also block norepinephrine and dopamine reuptake into the presynaptic neuron by competitive inhibition.

## Indications

- **ADHD**
- **Narcolepsy**

**Off-label**

- obesity, depression, chronic pain

## Pharmacokinetics

- Lipid-soluble form
- The peak response : 1-3 hours
- Metabolized: by CYP2D6
- The elimination is mainly via the urine

## Adverse Effects/Contraindications

**Common**

- Cardiovascular: Increased systolic arterial pressure
- Neurologic: Headache, insomnia
- Endocrine metabolic: Weight loss
- Gastrointestinal (GI): Dry mouth, decrease in appetite, weight loss, abdominal pain, nausea, diarrhea
- Psychiatric: Feeling nervous, mood swings

**Serious**

- Cardiovascular: Cardiomyopathy, myocardial infarction, peripheral vascular disease, Raynaud disease, sudden cardiac death
- Neurologic: Cerebrovascular accident, seizure
- Dermatologic: Stevens-Johnson syndrome, toxic epidermal necrolysis
- Immunologic: Hypersensitivity reaction
- Psychiatric: Psychotic disorder such as new or worsening psychotic or manic symptoms, behavior changes, or emotional lability

**Contraindications**

- Advanced arteriosclerosis
- Symptomatic cardiovascular disease
- Glaucoma
- History of drug abuse
- Hyperthyroidism
- Sudden death is one of the main concerns associated with CNS stimulant treatment

## Pearls

- *Monitoring*
- *It should not be prescribed to nursing women as it is excreted in human breast milk*
- *Evaluate ADHD patients for bipolar disorder risk factors before starting the treatment*
- *Monitor pediatric patients with new-onset or worsening aggressive behavior after starting the treatment*
- *Evaluate for any sign of peripheral vasculopathy such as Raynaud phenomenon, tics, and Tourette syndrome before and during treatment*
- *Abuse of this drugs became an epidemic during the last decade and is one of the main concerns*
- *Increased rates of depression, suicidal ideation, and attempts are seen more in the methamphetamine-abusing adolescent patient population*
- *The mechanism of toxicity is primarily related to excessive extracellular dopamine, norepinephrine, and serotonin*
- *The primary clinical syndrome involves prominent neurological and cardiovascular effects, but secondary complications can involve renal, muscle, pulmonary, and GI effects*
- *Hyperactivity, hyperthermia, tachycardia, tachypnea, mydriasis, tremors, seizures, and altered mental status are some of the most common signs and symptoms of amphetamine intoxication*
- *There is no antidote for amphetamine toxicity*

Stimulants

# Lisdexamfetamine (Vyvanse)

## Dosage Variations

- Capsules: 10mg, 20mg, 30mg, 40mg, 50mg, 60mg 70mg
- Chewable tablet: 10mg, 20mg, 30mg, 40mg, 50mg, 60mg

## Mechanism of Action

**Classification (CNS):** is a prodrug of dextroamphetamine, which is a noncatecholamine sympathomimetic amine with CNS stimulant activity. Dextroamphetamine is a known inhibitor of the dopamine transporter (DAT), noradrenaline transporter (NET) and vesicular monoamine transporter 2 (VMAT2), with a weaker affinity for the serotonin transporter (SERT). It is also a weak monoamine oxidase (MAO) inhibitor. Dextroamphetamine ultimately blocks the reuptake of norepinephrine and dopamine into the presynaptic neuron and increases catecholamine availability in the extracellular space.

## Indications

- **Attention Deficit Hyperactivity Disorder**
- **Binge Eating Disorder**
- **Prior to treatment, assess for presence of cardiac disease**
  - (eg, a careful history, family history of sudden death or ventricular arrhythmia, and physical exam)

## Pharmacokinetics

- Rapid absorption
- **Half-life elimination:** 10-13 hr
- **Excretion:** Urine
- plasma elimination half-life
- 8.6 to 9.5 hours in pediatric patients six to 12 years and 10 to 11.3 hours in healthy adults

## Adverse Effects/Contraindications

- Anorexia
- Insomnia
- Xerostomia
- Headache
- Upper abdominal pain
- Irritability
- Problem of growth and development, weight decreased (pediatric patients)
- Nausea
- Diarrhea
- Seizure
- Rash (pediatric patients)
- Hyperhidrosis
- Increased blood pressure
- Increased heart rate
- Dizziness
- Emotional lability
- Tremor
- Tics
- Vomiting

**Serious**

- Chest pain, sudden death (rare), myocardial infarction, palpitations, ventricular hypertrophy
- Cerebrovascular accident, Gilles de la Tourette syndrome
- Stevens-Johnson syndrome, toxic epidermal necrolysis due to drug

## Pearls

- *This medication has a high potential for abuse and misuse, which can lead to development of substance use disorder, including addiction*
- *Misuse and abuse of CNS stimulants can result in overdose and death*

Stimulants

# Methamphetamine (Desoxyn) HCL

## Dosage Variations

Methamphetamine can be ingested orally, through intravenous injection, smoked, and snorted

## Mechanism of Action

**Classification (Substituted Phenethylamine and Substituted Amphetamine):** Methamphetamine affects the central nervous system (CNS) by enhancing the release of monoamine neurotransmitters such as serotonin, dopamine, and norepinephrine. The use of methamphetamine can lead to many pharmacological effects because of its ability to use various molecular processes. Methamphetamine is highly lipid-soluble, which helps to be transferred relatively fast across the blood-brain barrier and has an immediate effect on the CNS.

## Indications

- **Attention Deficit Hyperactivity Disorder**

## Pharmacokinetics

- Half-Life: 4-5 hr
- Absorption: Rapid
- Metabolism: Liver
- Excretion: Urine, varies with pH

## Adverse Effects/Contraindications

People who use methamphetamine feel an acute, powerful short rush for about 5 to 30 minutes, which varies based on different routes of use

**Short-Term Effects**

- Decreased appetite
- Nausea
- Psychosis
- Tachycardia
- Hypertension
- Increased body temperature
- Panic attack
- Mydriasis (dilation of pupils)
- Disturbed sleep patterns
- Violent, bizarre, and erratic behavior
- Hallucinations and irritability
- Seizures, convulsions, and death from high doses

**Long-Term Effects**

- Long-lasting damage to the blood vessel of the heart and brain
- Lung, liver, and kidney damage
- Hypertension that can lead to heart attacks, strokes, and death
- Severe tooth degeneration
- In cases where the drug was sniffed, destruction of soft tissues in the nose
- In cases where the drug was smoked, respiratory problems
- In cases where the drug was injected, infectious diseases, cellulitis, and abscesses
- Weight loss and malnutrition
- Disorientation, apathy, confusion, and exhaustion
- Severe psychological dependence
- Psychosis
- Depression
- Damage to the brain structure similar to Alzheimer disease, epilepsy, and stroke

## Pearls

- *Users have different recognizable symptoms, for example, lack of sleep (insomnia), acute anxiety, agitation, and psychotic or violent behavior*
- *Tweaking — the last stage of methamphetamine misuse happens when the person who inappropriately uses methamphetamine becomes paranoid and irritable because of a lack of sleep for about 3 to 15 days*
- *Chronic meth users also usually show poor personal hygiene and sores on their bodies from picking at "crank bugs," unhealthy complexion, pallor, and tactile hallucinations that often occur in tweakers*
- *Methamphetamine users may develop cracked teeth because of extreme clenching of their jaw when they are high on methamphetamine*
- *It can cause physical and psychological dependence and increased tolerance*
- *Knowing the physical and behavioral symptoms of the methamphetamine overdose and diagnosis of the toxicity is essential for saving the patient's life*
- *Acute: When methamphetamine users experience an adverse reaction due to using a large amount of methamphetamine one time, it can be fatal.*
- *Prescribing this medication is limited due to its neurotoxic potential and risk of recreational use as a euphoriant*
- *Toxicity usually present with an altered mental status that can present as psychotic episodes, irritability, suicidal ideation, and rarely coma or seizures*
- *Chronic long-term use can also cause dental complications, significant weight loss, and skin problems such as sores and abscesses*

Stimulants

# Modafinil (Provigil)

## Dosage Variations

Modafinil is available exclusively in the form of 100 mg and 200 mg oral tablets; the usual dose is 200mg once daily. It is classified as a control substance class IV drug

## Mechanism of Action

**Classification (Class I Psychotropic):** The exact mechanism of action is unclear. Modafinil is known to be a weak inhibitor of dopamine reuptake, which may be its primary clinically important property. It has little to no in vivo affinity for the serotonin (5HT) or norepinephrine (NE) transporters. However, elevated concentrations of NE and 5HT in the prefrontal cortex and hypothalamus have been observed following modafinil administration, possibly as an indirect effect of increased extracellular dopamine. Modafinil activates glutamatergic circuits while inhibiting GABA. Modafinil has partial alpha 1B-adrenergic agonist effects by directly stimulating the receptors.

## Indications

**FDA-approved Indications**

- Narcolepsy
- Sleep Work Shift Disorder: First-line treatment
- Obstructive sleep apnea: Adjunct to continuous positive airway pressure (CPAP)

**Off-labeled Indications**

- Attention-deficit hyperactivity disorder
- Acute unipolar and bipolar depressive episodes
- Cocaine dependence
- Cancer-related fatigue
- Multiple sclerosis-related fatigues

## Pharmacokinetics

- Readily absorbed after oral administration
- Maximum plasma concentration is reached 2-4 hours after administration
- Hepatic metabolism via multiple pathways, including CYP3A4
- Excretion is urine
- The half-life of a single dose in healthy subjects is approximately 15 hours
- Severe renal and/or hepatic impairment is known to cause significantly increased steady-state drug concentrations

## Adverse Effects/Contraindications

- Common side effects are a headache, nausea, and decreased appetite, anxiety, insomnia, dizziness, diarrhea, and rhinitis
- Serious adverse effects, cases of Stevens-Johnson syndrome, toxic epidermal necrolysis, and drug rash with eosinophilia and systemic symptoms (DRESS)
- Assess the risk of potential abuse and use it with caution in patients with a history of drug abuse

**Contraindications**

- Dermatological reaction
- Angioedema and Anaphylaxis Reactions
- Multiorgan Hypersensitivity Reactions
- Persistent Sleepiness
- Cardiovascular disease
- Psychiatric disorders
- Tic disorders

## Pearls

- *Modafinil is a substrate of hepatic CYP3A4, a moderate inducer of CYP3A4, and a weak inhibitor of CYP2C19*
- *Case reports of modafinil overdose/toxicity are rare*
- *Modafinil is generally a well-tolerated stimulant, well-tolerated and carries a low potential for abuse*
- *Most of the reported cases of serious side effects have occurred within six weeks of drug initiation*
- *Overdose are relatively mild but may include hypertension, tachycardia, agitation, and/or psychosis*
- *Used cautiously in patients with structural cardiac disease, severe hepatic impairment, or a history of psychosis/mania*

Stimulants

# Atomoxetine (Strattera) HCL

## Dosage Variations

Atomoxetine is available in 10mg, 18mg, 25mg, 40mg, 60mg, 80mg, and 100mg capsules as a hydrochloride salt

## Mechanism of Action

**Classification (SNRIs):** Atomoxetine is a selective, presynaptic, norepinephrine reuptake inhibitor known as a NET inhibitor. Atomoxetine is the R(-) isomer. The R(-) isomer is an approximately nine times more potent norepinephrine reuptake inhibitor than the S(+) isomer.

## Indications

**FDA-approved Indication**

- Attention deficit hyperactivity disorder (ADHD)
- in adults and children over the age of 6

**Off-label Uses**

- Neurogenic orthostatic hypotension
- ADHD in adults with the comorbid partially responsive major depressive disorder
- Treatment-resistant administration

## Pharmacokinetics

- Atomoxetine is well-absorbed after oral administration and is minimally affected by food.
- It is metabolized predominantly through CYP2D6 enzymatic pathway
- The half-life is approximately 5 hours and may reach up to 24 hours in poor metabolizers
- Excreted primarily through the urine

## Adverse Effects/Contraindications

**Common Adverse Drug Reactions**

( Greater than 10)

- Headache (19)
- Insomnia (1 to 19)
- Hyperhidrosis (4 to 15)
- Xerostomia (17 to 35)
- Delayed ejaculation and priapism(8 to 21)
- Nausea (7 to 26)
- Decreased appetite (15 to 23)
- Abdominal pain (7 to 18)
- Vomiting (4 to 11)

**Adverse Drug Reactions (1 to 10)**

- Palpitations (3), cold extremities (1 to 3), prolonged QTc interval on ECG, increased diastolic blood pressure (5 to 9), greater than or equal to 15 mmHg), systolic hypertension (4 to 5), syncope (less than or equal to 3), orthostatic hypotension (less than or equal to 2), tachycardia (less than or equal to 2)
- Fatigue (6 to 10), dizziness (5 to 8), depression (4 to 7), disturbed sleep (3 to 7), irritability (5 to 6), jitteriness (2 to 5), abnormal dreams (4), chills (3), paresthesia (adults 3; postmarketing observation in children), anxiety (greater than or equal to 2), hostility (children and adolescents 2), emotional lability (1 to 2), agitation, restlessness, seizures
- Excoriation (2 to 4), rash (2), pruritus, urticaria,flushing (greater than or equal to 2)weight loss (2 to 7), hot flash (3), increased thirst (2), menstrual disease, dyspepsia (4), anorexia (3), dysgeusia, flatulence, urinary retention (1 to 6), dysmenorrhea (3), dysuria (2), pollakiuria, testicular pain, urinary frequency, tremor (1 to 5), muscle spasm, weakness, blurred vision (1 to 4), conjunctivitis (1 to 3)decreased libido (3), ejaculatory disorder (2 to 6)
- Hepatotoxicity (hepatocellular with marked increases in serum aminotransferase level)
- Women of childbearing age should use appropriate contraceptive measures as the adverse effects of atomoxetine have not been investigated thoroughly during pregnancy
- Women breastfeeding should exercise caution when taking atomoxetine as it is unknown if atomoxetine is excreted in breast milk
- Patients who are started on therapy should be observed closely for suicidality

## Pearls

- *Children and adolescents who start on atomoxetine require close monitoring for suicidal ideation and unusual changes in behavior*
- *Children should have their growth monitored*
- *All patients require monitoring for attention, hyperactivity, anxiety, aggression/hostility, and suicidal ideation*
- *Monitor for emergence of bipolar disorder/hypomania*
- *Tachycardia, nausea, vomiting, and hypertension were among the most common symptoms of toxicity*
- *Activated charcoal therapy and support of vital signs appear to be sufficient care during acute toxicity*

Stimulants

# Clonidine (Kapvay) HCL ER

## Mechanism of Action

## Dosage Variations

- Transdermal Patch (extended-release)
- Dosage: 0.1 mg/day, a mg/day, 0.3 mg/day. Change the patch every seven days
- Tablet (immediate-release)
- Dosage: 0.1 mg, 0.2 mg, 0.3 mg
- Tablet (extended-release)
- Dosage: 0.1 mg
- Injectable Solution
- Dosage: 100 mcg/ml, 500 mcg/ml

**Classification (Antihypertensives):** Clonidine hydrochloride is an imidazoline derivative that acts centrally on alpha-2 adrenergic as an agonist. The chemical name for clonidine is 2-((2,6-dichlorophenyl) amino)-2-imidazoline hydrochloride. As an alpha-adrenergic agonist in the nucleus tractus solitarii (NTS), clonidine excites a pathway that inhibits excitatory cardiovascular neurons. Clonidine has an alpha-antagonist effect in the posterior hypothalamus and medulla.

## Indications

- **Hypertension**
- **Treatment of attention deficit hyperactivity disorder (ADHD) in children**
- **Management of tics commonly found with Tourette syndrome**
- **Adjunct therapy for severing cancer-related pain**
- **Adjunct in neonatal opioid withdrawal syndrome**

**Off-label uses,** such as managing withdrawal symptoms from opioids, benzodiazepines, and alcohol and treating anxiety, insomnia, and post-traumatic stress disorder (PTSD)

## Pharmacokinetics

- Onset: <1 hr (2-4 hr peak effect in blood pressure)
- Duration: 6-10 hr
- Peak plasma time: 1-3 hr (immediate release); 7-8 hr (extended release)
- Metabolized in Liver
- Half-life: 6-20 hr
- Excretion: Urine

## Adverse Effects/Contraindications

**Common Reactions**

- Abdominal pain
- Headache
- Hypotension
- Fatigue
- Nausea
- Emotional instability
- Constipation
- Xerostomia
- Fever
- Diarrhea
- Sexual dysfunction
- Dizziness
- Sedation

**Serious Reactions**

- Angioedema
- Depression
- Hypersensitivity
- Atrioventricular (AV) block
- Bradycardia
- Syncope
- Severe hypotension

**Contraindications**

- Hypersensitivity to medication, class of alpha-2-agonist
- Dose adjustment is necessary for renal impairment, cardiovascular, bradycardia, hypotension, and severe coronary artery disease (CAD) patients
- Caution is necessary when treating patients with a history of depression, recent myocardial infarction (MI), and syncope
- It is also theoretically impair breast milk production because of decreased prolactin levels

## Pearls

- *Commonly used for withdrawal symptoms of opioid addiction, it has the potential to be a substance of misuse*
- *The potential of clonidine, when mixed with other benzodiazepines, opioids, or alcohol, can give the individual more potent drowsiness and further detachment from reality*
- *There is a case report recommending using naloxone to counter the sedative effects of Clonidine*

Stimulants

# Guanfacine (Intuniv) HCL ER

## Dosage Variations

Tablet (Tenex)

- 1mg
- 2mg

## Mechanism of Action

**Classification (Centrally Acting Alpha2A-Adrenergic Receptor Agonists):** Selective alpha2-adrenergic receptor agonist causing decreased sympathetic outflow and subsequent decrease in vasomotor tone and heart rate; may preferentially bind postsynaptic alpha2A adrenoreceptors in the prefrontal cortex, which may improve delay-related firing of prefrontal cortex neurons (as a result, behavioral inhibition may be affected); mechanism of action in ADHD is not known

## Indications

- **Hypertension**
- **Fragile X Syndrome (Orphan)**
- **ADHD**
- **in children**

**Off-label**

- Heroin Withdrawal
- Migraine Prophylaxis

## Pharmacokinetics

- Onset: 2 to 6 hrs
- Duration: 24 hr
- Half-life: 16 to 18 hrs
- Excretion: Urine
- Oxidized by CYP3A4

## Adverse Effects/Contraindications

- Cardiovascular: Bradycardia, palpitations, syncope, tachycardia, rebound hypertension, hypertensive encephalopathy
- CNS: Paresthesia, vertigo
- GI: Abdominal pain, constipation, diarrhea, dyspepsia, decreased appetite, nausea
- Liver/biliary: Abnormal LFTs
- Musculoskeletal: Arthralgia, leg cramps, leg pain, myalgia
- Psychiatric: Agitation, anxiety, confusion, depression, hallucinations, insomnia, nervousness
- Reproductive: Impotence
- Respiratory: Dyspnea
- Skin: Alopecia, dermatitis, exfoliative dermatitis, pruritus, rash
- Sensory: Blurred vision, alterations in taste
- Urinary: Nocturia, urinary frequency
- Other: Asthenia, chest pain, edema, malaise, tremor, headache
- Orthostatic hypotension
- Exfoliation
- Rash

**Contraindications**

- Hypersensitivity

## Pearls

- *Patients should not drive or operate heavy equipment until they know how they respond to guanfacine ER*
- *The safety and efficacy of the drug have not been established in children younger than six years of age*
- *Avoid alcohol*
- *Be sure to drink plenty of liquids and stay cool while you are taking this medication.*
- *Patients should be counselled regarding the risk of hypotension, bradycardia, and syncope*
- *Do not take with or immediately after a high-fat meal. High fat meals increase drug exposure*
- *Symptoms of overdose: drowsiness, lack of energy, slow heart rate, fainting, dizziness, blurred vision, smaller pupils*

## Dosage Variations

- Tablet (2.5mg, 5mg, 10mg)
- Capsule, extended-release (5mg, 10mg, 15mg, 20mg, 25mg, 30mg, 35mg, 40mg)

Stimulants

# Dexmethylphenidate (Focalin) HCL

## Mechanism of Action

**Classification (Stimulants):** The more pharmacologically active CNS stimulant of the d-threo-enantiomers; blocks reuptake of norepinephrine and dopamine, causing an increase of their release into the extraneuronal space. Methylphenidate inhibits dopamine and norepinephrine reuptake transporters in synapses, especially in the thalamus and striatum

## Indications

- **Attention deficit hyperactivity disorder - (ADHD)**

## Pharmacokinetics

- Onset of action: 12hr (extended release)
- Peak plasma time: 1-1.5 hr (Focalin XR: 2nd peak at 6.5 hr)
- Metabolites: Inactive
- Half-life: 2-4.5 hr (adults); 2-3 hr (children)
- Excretion: Urine
- CYP3A4 and CYP2D6

## Adverse Effects/Contraindications

**>10**

- Abdominal pain
- Headache
- Insomnia
- Restlessness
- Anxiety

**1-10**

- Anorexia
- Fever
- Dizziness
- Mood swings
- Nausea
- Pruritus
- Pharyngolaryngeal pain
- Irritability
- Depression
- Dyspepsia

**Postmarketing Reports**

- Anaphylaxis
- Hypersensitivity reactions
- Rhabdomyolysis
- Drowsiness
- Dyskinesia
- Tourette's syndrome (rare)
- Toxic psychosis
- Serotonin syndrome
- Abnormal liver function, ranging from transaminase elevation to severe hepatic injury

**Contraindications**

Hypersensitivity to methylphenidate; reactions may include angioedema and anaphylaxis

Notable tension and agitation, glaucoma, Tourette syndrome, motor tics, anxiety

## Pearls

- *Discontinue if no improvement after 1 month*
- *Do not use for depression, fatigue*
- *Use with caution in patients who use other sympathomimetic drugs*
- *Avoid alcohol*
- *This medication has a high potential for abuse and misuse, which can lead to development of substance use disorder, including addiction*

Stimulants

# Methylphenidate

(Concerta/ Daytrana Ritalin)

## Dosage Variations

- Tablet: Schedule II (5mg, 10mg, 20mg)
- Capsule, extended-release: Schedule II (10mg, 15mg, 20mg 25mg, 30mg, 35mg, 40mg, 45mg, 50mg, 55mg, 60mg, 70mg, 85mg)
- Oral solution: Schedule II (5mg/5mL, 10mg/5mL)

## Mechanism of Action

**Classification (CNS):** Methylphenidate blocks the reuptake of two neurotransmitters, norepinephrine (NE) and dopamine, in presynaptic neurons. More specifically, it inhibits the transporters of these neurotransmitters, increasing the concentration of dopamine and NE in the synaptic cleft. This creates its classic stimulant effect within the central nervous system (CNS), mainly in the prefrontal cortex.

## Indications

**FDA-approved**
- **Treating attention deficit hyperactivity disorder (ADHD)**
- **Children and adults and as a second-line treatment for narcolepsy in adults**

Off-label treatment for fatigue in patients with cancer, refractory depression in the geriatric population, apathy in Alzheimer disease, and enhancing cognitive performance (e.g., memory)

## Pharmacokinetics

- 1.9 hours for immediate-release tablets and 4.7 hours for extended-release tablets
- A majority of the drug is excreted in the urine
- Half Life is 2-3 hours (IR) and 3-5 hours (ER)
- Metabolized by the liver enzyme CYP2D6 (Cytochrome P450 2D6)

## Adverse Effects/Contraindications

- Insomnia and nervousness are the most commonly reported adverse effects in patients using methylphenidate
- Growth retardation (decreased height, weight, and bone marrow density) is observed when taken long-term in children
- Frequent side effects mainly involve the CNS (dizziness, headache, tics, restlessness/akathisia), gastrointestinal (nausea/vomiting, dry mouth, decreased appetite, weight loss, abdominal pain), and cardiovascular systems (tachycardia, and palpitations)
- Dermatologically, patients can complain of excessive sweating and ulceration of their digits
- Some patients may even develop blurry vision or decreased libido

**Contraindications**
- Patients must not use methylphenidate if they are currently on monoamine oxidase inhibitors (MAOIs)
- Children under the age of six should not be prescribed this medication as there are limited studies to prove its safety or benefit, and it could cause learning impairments

## Pearls

- *It has the potential risk of abuse, monitoring patients for signs of dependence and or abuse while on therapy*
- *A complete blood count with differential should be obtained periodically for those on methylphenidate*
- *The main vitals to note at each visit are blood pressure and heart rate, especially in patients with underlying hypertension, heart failure, a recent MI, or ventricular arrhythmia, as slight elevations can occur with methylphenidate use*
- *Clinicians should screen for symptoms of depression, agitation, aggressiveness, new-onset or pre-existing psychosis or mania, and suicidality as these can be worsened when initially starting methylphenidate*
- *The first step in a medication overdose is to immediately contact a poison control center for the appropriate management steps*
- *Doses that exceed 60 mg of the IR (immediate-release) formulation or 120 mg of the ER (extended-release) formulation can be considered toxic*

Stimulants

# Benzphetamine HCL (Didrex/ Recede)

## Dosage Variations

Tablet: Schedule III

- 25mg (Regimex)
- 50mg (Didrex)

## Mechanism of Action

**Classification (Sympathomimetic Amines):** Benzphetamine, a phenylalkylamin, is related to amphetamine both chemically and pharmacologically. It is an anorectic agent indicated in the management of exogenous obesity as a short term adjunct (a few weeks) in a regimen of weight reduction based on caloric restriction. Amphetamines stimulate noepinephrine and dopamine release in nerve endings in the lateral hypothalamic feeding centre, decreasing appetite. This release is mediated by the binding of benzphetamine to centrally located adrenergic receptors.

## Indications

- **Obesity**
  - as a short term (a few weeks)
- **Adjunct in a regimen of weight reduction based on caloric restriction**
  - Patients with an initial body mass index (BMI) of ≥30 kg/m² who have not responded to appropriate weight reducing regimen (diet and/or exercise) alone

## Pharmacokinetics

- Metabolized by cytochrome P450 enzymes
- Excretion: 5-30% unchanged in urine, highly dependent on pH
- Readily absorbed from the gastro-intestinal tract and buccal mucosa
- Half Life: 16-31

## Adverse Effects/Contraindications

Contraindications

- Advanced arteriosclerosis
- Symptomatic cardiovascular disease including arrhythmias
- Hyperthyroidism
- Moderate to severe hypertension
- Hypersensitivity to sympathomimetic amines
- Glaucoma
- Agitated state
- History of drug abuse
- Pregnancy/lactation; women planning to get pregnant
- Do not use in combination with other anorectic agents including prescription, OTC, or herbal
- Valvular heart disease associated with use of some anorectics (no cases reported with benzphetamine monotherapy)
- Not recommended for patients who used any anorectic agents within prior year

- Abdominal pain
- Blood pressure increase
- Constipation
- Diarrhea
- Dizziness
- Dry mouth
- Headache

- Insomnia
- Ischemic cardiac events associated with chronic amphetamine use
- Libido changes
- Nausea
- Palpitations
- Psychotic episodes (rare)
- Restlessness
- Tachycardia
- Tremor

## Pearls

- *Excreted in human milk; mothers taking amphetamines should be advised to refrain from nursing*
- *Limit caffeine intake*

Section 6

# Anxiolytics

Anxiolytics (Long Acting)

# Buspirone (Buspar)

## Dosage Variations

- Oral tablets in 5mg, 7.5mg, 10mg, 15mg, and 30mg oral tablets
- The maximum daily dosage is 60 mg per day

## Mechanism of Action

**Classification (Anxiolytic Drug):** Buspirone is classified in the azapirone drug class. It has a strong affinity for serotonin 5HT1a receptors, where it acts as a partial agonist, which some researchers believe produces the preponderance of clinical effects. It also has a weak affinity for serotonin 5HT2 receptors and acts as a weak antagonist on dopamine D2 autoreceptors. There is no effect on benzodiazepine GABA receptors.

## Indications

**FDA-approved**

- **Anxiety disorders**

**Off-label**

- Augmentation of unipolar depression
- Buspirone combined with melatonin can treat major depressive disorder (MDD) and promote neurogenesis

## Pharmacokinetics

- Buspirone is rapidly absorbed and undergoes extensive first-pass metabolism
- Metabolized primarily by oxidation by CYP3A4
- The half-life of unchanged buspirone is approximately 2 to 3 hours
- It is excreted in the urine

## Adverse Effects/Contraindications

- Dizziness is a common side effect
- Central nervous system (CNS): Abnormal dreams, ataxia, confusion, dizziness, drowsiness, excitement, headache, nervousness, numbness, outbursts of anger, paresthesia
- Ophthalmic: Blurred vision
- Otic: Tinnitus
- Cardiovascular: Chest pain
- Respiratory: Nasal congestion
- Dermatologic: Diaphoresis, skin rash
- Gastrointestinal: Diarrhea, nausea, sore throat
- Neuromuscular and skeletal: Musculoskeletal pain, tremor, weakness
- Hepatic: isolated cases of serum enzyme elevations without jaundice

**Contraindications**

- History of hypersensitivity reaction with Buspirone in the past
- Avoid the use of monoamine oxidase inhibitors (MAOI) within 14 days before or after Buspirone therapy. Due to the risk of developing serotonin syndrome and/or elevated blood pressure

## Pearls

- *Typically, it is used as a second-line agent behind selective serotonin reuptake inhibitors(SSRIs) when a patient does not respond to or cannot tolerate the side effects of SSRIs. Encourage patients to stay consistent with their medication schedule and whether they take it with food*
- *Healthcare providers should closely monitor signs and symptoms of anaphylaxis, akathisia, and serotonin syndrome*
- *Alcohol use can worsen any CNS sedation, and its use requires strict monitoring as well*
- *Buspirone has also been used as an augmentation agent to reduce SSRI's sexual side effects*
- *It is important to note that no specific antidote is known for Buspirone*

Anxiolytics (Long Acting)

# Chlordiazepoxide (Librium)

## Dosage Variations

- Oral Capsule available in 5mg, 10mg, and 25mg and as an injectable with a concentration of 100mg / 5ml
- It is usually in the form of a gelatin capsule, and storage should be at 68F to 77F (20C to 25C).

## Mechanism of Action

**Classification (Benzodiazepines):** Chlordiazepoxide has anti-anxiety, sedative, appetite-stimulating, and weak analgesic actions. It binds to benzodiazepine receptors at the GABA-A ligand-gated chloride channel complex and enhances GABA's inhibitory effects. Also, it increases chloride conductance through GABA-regulated channels.

## Indications

**FDA approved**
- Mild-moderate to severe anxiety disorder
- Preoperative apprehension and anxiety
- Withdrawal symptoms of acute alcohol use disorder
- Pediatric patients
    - Greater than six years old for anxiety

**Off-label:** Catatonia

## Pharmacokinetics

- Onset: 1-5 min (IV)
- Duration: 15-60 min (IV)
- CYP2C19
- Half-life: 6-25 hr (normal liver and renal function); 5-30 hr (end-stage renal disease); 30-63 hr (liver cirrhosis)
- Excretion: Urine

## Adverse Effects/Contraindications

- Common side effects include fatigue, sedation, depression, dizziness, ataxia, slurred speech, weakness, confusion, forgetfulness, nervousness, hyperexcitability, and pain at the injection site
- Some of the rare side effects include mania, weight gain, hallucination, hypotension, skin eruptions, menstrual irregularity, dry mouth, and hyper-salivation
- Life-threatening side effects are blood dyscrasias, renal dysfunction, hepatic dysfunction, and respiratory depression, particularly when taken with CNS depressants in overdose

**Contraindications**
- It is not recommended for a pregnant patient or planning to get pregnant due to the potential risk of congenital anomalies, especially during the first trimester
- Chlordiazepoxide may reduce the mental and physical abilities needed for the performance of some tasks, including driving a vehicle or operating heavy machinery
- It may diminish mental alertness in children

## Pearls

- *There is a reported risk of dependence with long term use*
- *Patients on anticoagulation should require monitoring for possible blood coagulation*
- *Patients with porphyria also need monitoring because of possible porphyria exacerbation*
- *In cases of chlordiazepoxide overdose or toxicity, the patient may present with confusion, diminished reflexes, comatose, or somnolent*
- *Patient respiration, blood pressure, and pulse must have regular monitoring*

## Dosage Variations

- Tablet: (2mg, 5mg, 10mg)
- Oral solution:(1mg/1mL, 5mg/mL)
- rectal gel (2.5mg/0.5mL, 10mg/2mL, 20mg/4mL)
- Injectable solution: Schedule IV (5mg/mL)
- Intramuscular device: Schedule IV (5mg/mL)
- intranasal spray (Valtoco): (5mg , 7.5mg, 10mg/0.1mL)

Anxiolytics (Long Acting)

# Diazepam (Valium)

## Mechanism of Action

**Classification (CNS):** Benzodiazepines exert their effects by facilitating the activity of gamma-aminobutyric acid(GABA) at various sites. Specifically, benzodiazepines bind at an allosteric site at the interface between the alpha and gamma subunits on GABA-A receptor chloride ion channels. The allosteric binding of diazepam at the GABA-A receptor increases the frequency at which the chloride channel opens, leading to an increased conductance of chloride ions. This shift in charge leads to a hyperpolarization of the neuronal membrane and reduced neuronal excitability.

## Indications

- **Anxiety disorders**
- **Alcohol detoxification**
- **Acute recurrent seizures**
- **Severe muscle spasms and spasticity associated with neurologic disorders**
- **In acute alcohol withdrawal**
- **Treats anxiety and sleep disorders**
  - Availability that can reverse over sedation in cases of benzodiazepine intoxication

**Off-label (non-FDA approved)** use for diazepam includes sedation in the ICU and short-term treatment of spasticity in children with cerebral palsy

## Pharmacokinetics

- Metabolized by hepatic P450 enzymes CYP2C19, CYP3A4
- Half life: 20-70 hr (active metabolite); 49.2 hr (10-mg intranasal dose)
- Excretion: Urine

## Adverse Effects/Contraindications

- The adverse reactions of diazepam include CNS and respiratory depression, dependence, and benzodiazepine withdrawal syndrome

**Serious adverse effects of diazepam include:**
- Respiratory depression
- Suicidality
- Dependency and abuse
- Withdrawal symptoms
- Cardiovascular collapse
- Bradycardia
- Hypotension
- Syncope
- Paradoxical CNS stimulation

**Common adverse effects of diazepam include:**
- Sedation
- Fatigue
- Confusion
- Anterograde amnesia
- Depression
- Ataxia
- Irritability
- Disinhibition
- Local injection site reaction
- Headache
- Tremor
- Dystonia
- Urinary retention
- Incontinence
- Nausea
- Constipation
- Diplopia
- Libido changes
- Rash
- Menstrual irregularities
- ALT and/or AST elevation

**Contraindications**
- Contraindicated in patients under six months of age
- Other contraindications to diazepam include patients with severe respiratory insufficiency, myasthenia gravis, sleep apnea syndrome, and severe hepatic insufficiency
- It is permissible in patients with open-angle glaucoma receiving appropriate therapy but is contraindicated in acute narrow-angle glaucoma
- The persistent and chronic use of benzodiazepines, including diazepam, can lead to physical dependence if used more frequently than recommended

**US Boxed Warning**
- The use of benzodiazepines and opioids may result in respiratory depression, profound sedation, coma, and death

## Pearls

- *Monitoring respiratory and cardiovascular status, blood pressure, heart rate, and anxiety symptoms in patients taking diazepam is crucial*
- *With long-term use, monitor liver enzymes, CBC, and for signs of propylene glycol toxicity, including serum creatinine, BUN, serum lactate, and osmolality gap*
- *Monitor the depth of sedation*
- *There is a potential of overdose when combined with opioids, alcohol, or other centrally acting agents*
- *In cases of severe overdose, symptoms manifest as ataxia, diminished reflexes, hypotonia, hypotension, respiratory depression, coma (rarely), and death (rarely)*
- *Caution Renal and Hepatic Impairment*

## Dosage Variations

Capsule: Schedule IV
(15mg, 30mg)

Anxiolytics (Long Acting)

# Flurazepam (Dalmane)

## Mechanism of Action

**Classification (CNS):** Flurazepam enhances the effects of gamma-aminobutyric acid (GABA), which is the primary inhibitory neurotransmitter in the central nervous system. GABA reduces the activity of neurons to which it binds. Benzodiazepines like flurazepam bind to specific sites on the GABA-A receptor complex and enhance the binding of GABA to its receptor. This enhances the inhibitory effect of GABA, leading to increased neuronal inhibition.

## Indications

- **Insomnia**
- **Anxiety**

## Pharmacokinetics

- Metabolism: Liver : CYP3A4
- Excretion: Urine
- Half-life elimination: 48-120 h
- Absorbed well orally

## Adverse Effects/Contraindications

**Common**
- Ataxia
- Dizziness
- Drowsiness
- Lethargy
- Light-headedness

**Less Common**
- Chest pain, palpitations
- Headache, irritability, nervousness, weakness
- GI complaints
- Myalgia
- GU complaints

**Rare**
- Elevations of AST, ALT, bilirubin (T&D), alk phos

**Black Box Warnings**
- Concomitant use of benzodiazepines and opioids may result in profound respiratory depression, coma, and death; administer concomitantly when there are no alternative options; limit dosages and durations to minimum required; monitor for signs and symptoms of respiratory depression and sedation

**Contraindications**
- Documented hypersensitivity

## Pearls

- *Flurazepam is primarily indicated for the short-term treatment of insomnia*
- *Abrupt discontinuation should be avoided to prevent withdrawal symptoms*
- *Can cause anterograde amnesia, so patients should be cautioned against engaging in activities that require complete mental alertness, such as driving or operating machinery.*
- *It should be used for short periods only (generally 7 to 10 days), as long-term use can lead to tolerance, dependence, and withdrawal symptoms*
- *Caution should be exercised when prescribing to elderly patients due to the increased risk of falls, cognitive impairment, and accumulation of the drug in the system.*
- *Alcohol should be avoided while taking flurazepam, as it can increase the sedative effects and lead to excessive drowsiness and impaired coordination*

## Dosage Variations

- Tablet (0.25mg, 0.5mg, 1mg, 2mg)
- Tablet, extended-release: (0.5mg, 1mg, 2mg, 3mg)
- Tablet, orally disintegrating: (0.25mg, 0.5mg, 1mg, 2mg)
- Oral solution: (1 mg/mL)

### Anxiolytics (Intermediate Acting)

# Alprazolam (Xanax)

## Mechanism of Action

**Classification (Benzodiazepines):** Alprazolam belongs to a class of psychoactive medications called benzodiazepines. Benzodiazepines bind to the GABA-A receptor. This receptor is comprised of five subunits, e.g., alpha, beta, gamma, delta, epsilon, rho, etc. A common GABA-A receptor in the CNS is comprised of two alpha-1 subunits, two beta-2 subunits, and one gamma-2 subunit.

## Indications

- **Panic disorders**
- **Anxiety disorders**

**Off-label**

- Insomnia
- Premenstrual syndrome
- Depression

## Pharmacokinetics

- It is rapidly absorbed after oral administration
- Peak plasma concentration at 1 to 2 hours
- Metabolized in the liver
- Cytochrome P450 3A4 (CYP3A4)
- Its metabolites are filtered out by the kidneys and excreted in the urine
- Half-life of alprazolam is about 11.2 hours in healthy adults

## Adverse Effects/Contraindications

- Drowsiness
- Tiredness
- Dizziness
- Sleep problems (insomnia)
- Memory problems
- Poor balance or coordination
- Slurred speech
- Trouble concentrating
- Irritability
- Diarrhea
- Constipation
- Increased sweating
- Headache
- Nausea
- Vomiting
- Upset stomach
- Blurred vision
- Appetite or weight changes
- Swelling of hands or feet
- Muscle weakness
- Dry mouth
- Stuffy nose
- Loss of interest in sex
- Worsening depression
- Hypomania
- Decreased mental alertness
- Neonatal sedation and withdrawal syndrome

*Medications known to impact alprazolam include azole antifungals (ketoconazole), cimetidine, certain anti-depressants (fluoxetine, fluvoxamine, and nefazodone), macrolide antibiotics (clarithromycin), rifamycins (rifampin), St. John's wort, seizure medications (carbamazepine, phenytoin), antihistamines and muscle relaxants*

## Pearls

- *Alprazolam should be avoided if possible by anyone with pulmonary disease*
- *Using alprazolam with CNS depressants, especially opioids, increases the risk of respiratory depression, low blood pressure, and death*
- *Alprazolam has also been subject to misuse for recreational purposes because of its disinhibition, euphoria, and anxiolytic effects*
- *Patients should also have monitoring for orthostasis, excessive sedation, and a periodic basic metabolic panel*
- *Liver function tests and complete blood counts also require observation during chronic therapy*
- *Benzodiazepines can cross the placenta, so clinicians should observe newborns for signs/symptoms of sedation, respiratory depression, feeding problems, and neonatal withdrawal syndrome for infants having in-utero exposure to alprazolam*
- *It is recommended to taper to discontinue alprazolam gradually*
- *In alprazolam overdose cases, respiration, blood pressure, and pulse rate require monitoring*
- *Drugs that are potent inhibitors of CYP3A may increase plasma concentrations of alprazolam, resulting in increased adverse events*

Anxiolytics (Intermediate Acting)

# Clonazepam (Klonopin)

## Dosage Variations

- Immediate-release tablet of 0.5mg, 1mg, 2mg
- Orally disintegrated tablets (ODT) of 0.125mg, 0.25mg, 0.5mg, 1mg, and 2mg strength

## Mechanism of Action

**Classification (Benzodiazepines):** Clonazepam is a highly potent long-acting benzodiazepine. Clonazepam exerts pharmacological effects by acting as a positive allosteric modulator of GABA-A receptors. The GABA-A receptor is a ligand-gated chloride ion selective channel whose endogenous ligand is GABA (gamma-aminobutyric acid). Benzodiazepines facilitate GABA-A action by increasing the frequency of chloride channel opening resulting in hyperpolarization of the neurons and reduced firing, thus producing calming effects on the brain by decreasing the excitability of neurons.

## Indications

- **Status Epilepticus**
- **Panic disorders with or without agoraphobia**
- **Acute mania**

***Off-label*** *use as monotherapy or adjunctive therapy to treat mania, restless leg syndrome, insomnia, tardive dyskinesia, and REM sleep behavior disorder, burning mouth syndrome*

## Pharmacokinetics

- Onset: 20-40 min
- Peak plasma time: 1-4 hr; 5-7 days (steady state)
- Metabolized by CYP3A4
- Half-life: 17-60 hr (adults); 22-33 hr (children)
- Excretion: Urine

## Adverse Effects/Contraindications

- The most commonly associated with lethargy, fatigue, sedation, drowsiness, and motor impairment (impaired coordination, impaired balance, dizziness)
- Less Common Side Effects can cause blurred vision, confusion, irritability, loss of libido, lack of motivation, psychomotor agitation, hallucination, worsening of depression, short-term memory loss, and anterograde amnesia, especially with high doses
- Occasional adverse effects of clonazepam include personality changes, behavioral disturbance, ataxia, increased frequency of seizures, thrombocytopenia, and dysphoria
- Rare but important side effects of clonazepam include paradoxical disinhibition, i.e., excitement, rage, and impulsive behavior
- Concurrent use of benzodiazepines and opioids may result in sedation, respiratory depression, coma, and death

## Pearls

- *Monitor Complete Blood Count, Renal, and Liver Function*
- *It can cause worsening of seizures*
- *The use of benzodiazepines, including clonazepam, has the potential for misuse and addiction*
- *Abrupt discontinuation should be avoided*
- *Respiratory compromise exercise extreme caution when taking clonazepam*
- *Impaired cognitive and motor performance can be a potential effects*
- *Increased risk of depression, suicidal behavior and thinking*
- *Strongly avoid alcohol use*
- *Monitoring for misuse/abuse*
- *Any level over 0.08 mcg/mL is considered toxic*

Anxiolytics (Intermediate Acting)

# Lorazepam (Ativan)

## Dosage Variations

- Orally tablet (0.5mg, 1mg, 2mg)
- Oral concentrate solution 2mg/mL,
- Intravenous(IV) or intramuscular(IM) injection (2mg/mL solution and 4mg/mL solution)
- The onset of its action is 1 to 3 minutes if administered IV and 15 to 30 minutes if administered IM.

## Mechanism of Action

**Classification (Benzodiazepines):** Lorazepam binds to benzodiazepine receptors on the postsynaptic GABA-A ligand-gated chloride channel neuron at several sites within the central nervous system (CNS). It enhances the inhibitory effects of GABA, which increases the conductance of chloride ions in the cell. This shift in chloride ions results in hyperpolarization and stabilization of the cellular plasma membrane.

## Indications

**FDA-approved Indications**

- Short-term (4 months) relief of anxiety symptoms related to anxiety disorders
- Anxiety-associated insomnia
- Anesthesia premedication in adults to relieve anxiety or to produce sedation/amnesia
- Treatment of status epilepticus

**Off-label (non-FDA-approved) Indications**

- Rapid tranquilization of the agitated patient
- Alcohol withdrawal delirium
- Alcohol withdrawal syndrome
- Insomnia
- Panic disorder
- Delirium
- Chemotherapy-associated anticipatory nausea and vomiting (adjunct or breakthrough)
- Psychogenic catatonia
- Vertigo

## Pharmacokinetics

- Hepatic metabolism
- Absorbed in the GI tract
- Metabolized in Liver
- Half-life: 18 hr (children 2-12 years); 42 hr (neonates); 28 hr (adolescents); 12 hr (tablets, adults); 20.2 hr (capsules, adults)
- Excretion: Urine

## Adverse Effects/Contraindications

- Respiratory depression
- Respiratory failure
- Seizures
- Suicidality
- Dependency and abuse
- Tachycardia
- Hypotension
- Syncope
- Blood dyscrasias
- Jaundice
- Paradoxical reaction; hyperactive and aggressive behavior
- Gangrene (intra-arterial)
- Cognitive deficits
- Behavioral changes
- Paradoxical agitation
- Sedation
- Dizziness
- Asthenia
- Ataxia
- Local injection site reaction
- Respiratory depression
- Hypoventilation with IV use
- Hypotension
- Fatigue
- Amnesia
- Confusion
- Disinhibition
- Irritability
- Libido changes
- Menstrual irregularities
- Diplopia
- Dysarthria
- Appetite changes
- Constipation
- Incontinence
- Urinary retention
- Dystonia
- AST and ALT elevation

**Contraindications**

Contraindicated to use in neonates or premature infants, in patients with severe respiratory impairment

## Pearls

- *Monitor respiratory and cardiovascular status, blood pressure, and heart rate*
- *Monitor and adjust the dose of lorazepam according to the Clinical Institute Withdrawal Assessment for Alcohol–Revised (CIWA-Ar) protocol*
- *It should not be first-line agents for anxiety and other psychiatric disorder symptoms in the first and third trimesters of pregnancy*
- *Monitor for improvement in anxiety by using a validated scoring system like Hamilton Anxiety Scale*
- *Lorazepam can cause CNS and respiratory depression in overdose*
- *In rare instances, lorazepam can cause acute liver injury(cholestatic pattern)*
- *It can lead to hypotension, ataxia, confusion, coma, extreme drowsiness, muscle weakness, and death*
- *Flumazenil is an antidote for benzodiazepine toxicity*
- *It is not extensively metabolized by cytochrome P450 (CYP) enzymes; CYP enzymes are not the primary route of metabolism for lorazepam*
- *Withdrawal symptoms if abruptly discontinued after long-term use*

## Dosage Variations

Capsule of 10 mg, 15mg, or 30mg or tablet of 15mg. No dose adjustments are needed for patients with hepatic or renal impairments

Anxiolytics (Intermediate Acting)

# Oxazepam (Serax)

## Mechanism of Action

**Classification (CNS):** The most prescribed medications for the treatment of insomnia and anxiety

## Indications

**FDA-approved**

- Treatment of alcohol withdrawal and the management of anxiety disorders
    - Not FDA-approved for use in children under the age of six due to the risk of respiratory arrest.
- Recommended agent in patients who have difficulties remaining asleep
    - In contrast to drugs helping to initiate sleep

## Pharmacokinetics

- Half-life elimination: 2.8-5.7 hr
- Peak plasma time: 3 hr
- Excretion: Urine
- Primarily metabolized in the liver

## Adverse Effects/Contraindications

- Adverse effects may include sedation, fatigue, depression, confusion, memory impairment, dizziness, ataxia, slurred speech, hyper-excitability, nervousness, and weakness
- Less frequently encountered adverse effects may involve hypotension, hallucinations, mania, dry mouth, hypersalivation, edema, leukopenia, decreased libido, incontinence, rash, menstrual irregularities, jaundice, and diplopia
- Severe adverse effects of Oxazepam include respiratory depression and neonatal abstinence syndrome

**Contraindications**

- Patients taking Oxazepam for insomnia should avoid caffeine-containing products as they may decrease the efficacy of the drug
- It is also not recommended for those who suffer from sleep apnea
- Oxazepam may also cross the placenta and be excreted into breastmilk; thus, it is not a recommended pharmaceutical therapy in pregnant or nursing women
- Oxazepam use is not recommended for geriatric patients due to increased risk of dependence and cognitive impairment as well as falls

## Pearls

- *It is critical to monitor cardiovascular and respiratory status and hemodynamic stability and vital signs*
- *Toxicity can present as other conditions—especially in long-term Oxazepam use—so it is crucial to collect appropriate labs such as CBC, BUN/creatinine, and other serum values when deemed necessary*
- *It is the least sedating among all benzodiazepines due to slower absorption*

## Anxiolytics (Intermediate Acting)

# Temazepam (Restoril)

### Dosage Variations

- Available in liquid, gel, or powder forms and packaged in either hard or soft capsules
- The available dosage strengths of temazepam include 7.5mg, 10mg, 15mg, 20mg, and 30mg
- Capsules are formulated in 7.5mg, 15mg, 22.5mg, and 30mg for oral administration

## Mechanism of Action

**Classification (Benzodiazepines):** Temazepam induces central nervous system (CNS) depression by affecting the limbic, thalamic, and hypothalamic regions. Temazepam exerts its pharmacological effects, including drowsiness, hypnosis, skeletal muscle relaxation, anticonvulsant action, and anxiolysis, by binding to benzodiazepine receptors. These receptors constitute several GABA-A receptor subtypes, with a particular affinity for α1 subunits.

## Indications

- **Insomnia and other sleep-related issues**
  - including frequent awakenings during the night or early in the morning
- **Maintaining sleep**
  - although its impact on the delay in sleep onset is relatively modest

***Off-Label Uses*** can be beneficial in addressing sleep disruptions associated with jet lag. It is also capable of relaxing skeletal muscles

## Pharmacokinetics

- Metabolized by CYP3A4 (minor), glucuronic acid conjugation
- Metabolites: Inactive
- Half-life elimination: 9.5-12.4 hr
- Excretion: Urine

## Adverse Effects/Contraindications

**Adverse Drug Reactions**

- Cardiovascular system included palpitations, whereas gastrointestinal symptoms included xerostomia, dysgeusia, emesis, diarrhea, epigastric discomfort, and constipation.
- Neurological symptoms included headache, disorientation, drowsiness, dizziness, giddiness, unsteadiness, anterograde amnesia, and paresthesia

**Contraindications**

- Temazepam is contraindicated in pregnancy, as it is classified as an FDA pregnancy category X drug

**Box Warnings**

- Increased risks of severe sedation and potentially fatal respiratory depression when combined with opioids
- Intravenous administration is the main method of abuse for temazepam capsules

**Precautions**

- The use of temazepam should be minimized or entirely avoided in individuals with severe motor coordination impairment, acute intoxication with alcohol, opioids, or other psychoactive substances, sleep apnea, myasthenia gravis, acute narrow-angle glaucoma, clinically significant major depressive disorder with suicidal ideation, renal and hepatic insufficiency, hypersensitivity, or allergy to any benzodiazepines

## Pearls

- *It can adversely impact social and mental health and cause violent outbursts at home and in public and psychological disorders, including paranoia and other irrational behaviors*
- *A multi approach should be considered to address sleep problems effectively and choose the optimal treatment option*
- *Deaths from self-poisoning with temazepam alone or in combination with other substances were shown to be more common*

Section 6

# Anxiolytics

## Short Acting

## Dosage Variations

Oral syrup: Schedule IV

- 2mg/mL (generic)

Injectable solution: Schedule IV

- 1mg/mL (generic)
- 5mg/mL (generic, Seizalam)

Anxiolytics (Short Acting)

# Midazolam (Versed)

## Mechanism of Action

**Classification (Benzodiazepines):** Midazolam has poor oral absorption and has an elimination half-life of 1.5 to 2.5 hours. Midazolam converts into its active metabolite alpha-1 hydroxy midazolam, which contributes to 10% of drug action. Midazolam metabolism occurs via hepatic CYP450 enzymes and glucuronide conjugation.

## Indications

- **Acute seizures**
- **Status epilepticus**
- **Anxiolysis and hypnosis**
    - during the maintenance phase of general anesthesia

## Pharmacokinetics

- Onset: 15-20 min (IM, PO); 3-5 min (IV)
- Metabolized by liver via CYP3A4
- Half-life: 2-6 hr
- Excretion: Urine

## Adverse Effects/Contraindications

- Common adverse effects associated with Midazolam use are hiccoughs, cough, nausea, and vomiting
- Thrombophlebitis, thrombosis, and pain on injection are other adverse effects
- Can cause nanterograde amnesia, drowsiness, ataxia, falls, and confusion in the elderly
- Residual hangover effects can happen with nighttime administration of Midazolam, which can impair the cognitive and psychomotor abilities, which can result in falls in elderly and impaired coordination during driving
- Hypotension and tachycardia can occur with rapid intravenous administration
- Concomitant use of midazolam with other CNS depressants can result in severe respiratory depression and death even at therapeutic doses
- Long-term use of midazolam is associated with lasting memory deficits, which are only partially reversible after discontinuing the drug
- For pregnant women, the administration of the drug in the third trimester causes benzodiazepine withdrawal syndrome in the neonate
- The use of midazolam includes acute angle-closure glaucoma, hypotension, and shock
- Careful dose adjustment is necessary in cases of kidney and liver diseases, alcohol, and drug-dependent individuals
- Extra precautions should be taken in critically ill individuals as dose accumulation can occur

## Pearls

- *Frequent monitoring of blood levels of midazolam and its metabolites is a requirement during the treatment of midazolam overdose*
- *Levels of midazolam and its metabolites can be measurable in blood, plasma, and serum*
- *Toxicity with midazolam is rare but can happen when combined with other CNS depressants like alcohol, opioids, and other tricyclic antidepressants*
- *The risk increases with intravenous administration and in elderly individuals with COPD*
- *Symptoms of overdose include ataxia, nystagmus, hypotension, slurred speech, slurred speech, impaired motor coordination, coma, and death*
- *Flumazenil is the antidote for midazolam toxicity*

Anxiolytics (Short Acting)

# Triazolam (Halcion)

## Dosage Variations

Tablet: Schedule IV (0.125mg ,0.25mg)

## Mechanism of Action

**Classification (CNS):** Depresses all levels of CNS (eg, limbic and reticular formation), possibly by increasing membrane permeability to chloride ions, which in turn increases the inhibitory activity of GABA on neuronal excitability.

## Indications

- **Insomnia**

**Dosage Modifications**

- Hepatic impairment: Administer a lower dose; avoid use in cirrhosis

## Pharmacokinetics

- Half-Life: 1.5-5.5 hr
- Peak plasma time: 0.5-2 hr
- Onset of action: 15-30 min
- Duration: 6-7 hr
- Peak plasma concentration: 1-6 ng/mL
- Metabolism: CYP3A4, glucuronic acid conjugation
- Excretion: Urine

## Adverse Effects/Contraindications

- Drowsiness
- Headache
- Dizziness
- Nervousness
- Ataxia
- Lightheadedness
- N/V

- Anterogade amnesia
- Paradoxical reactions
- Travelers amnesia- especially if combined with EtOH
- Confusion
- Cramps
- Fatigue
- Memory impairment
- Depression
- Visual disturbance
- Xerostomia
- Anterograde amnesia
- Dreaming/nightmares
- Confusion

**Contraindications**

- Documented hypersensitivity
- Acute alcohol intoxication
- Myasthenia gravis (allowable in limited circumstances)
- Narrow angle glaucoma (questionable)
- Severe respiratory depression
- Depressed neuroses, psychotic reactions
- IV use in shock, coma, depressed respiration, patients who recently received other respiratory depressants

**Black Box Warnings**

- Risks from concomitant use with opioids
- Concomitant use of benzodiazepines and opioids may result in profound sedation, respiratory depression, coma, and death
- Reserve concomitant prescribing of these drugs for use in patients for whom alternative treatment options are inadequate

**Addiction, abuse, and misuse**

- Addiction, abuse, and misuse, which can lead to overdose and death

## Pearls

- *There are no data on presence of drug in human milk or effects on milk production; there are reports of central nervous system depression (sedation, respiratory depression), withdrawal symptoms, and feeding problems in infants who are breastfed by mothers taking benzodiazepines*

ISBN 978-1-7369010-4-5
9 781736 901045

Made in the USA
Monee, IL
26 April 2026

49012547R00049